UNEQUAL PARTNERS

User groups and community care

Marian Barnes, Stephen Harrison,
Maggie Mort and Polly Shardlow

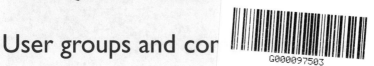

The POLICY
P~P
PRESS

First published in Great Britain in 1999 by

The Policy Press
University of Bristol
34 Tyndall's Park Road
Bristol BS8 1PY
UK
Tel no +44 (0)117 973 8797
Fax no +44 (0)117 973 7308
E-mail tpp@bristol.ac.uk
http://www.bristol.ac.uk/Publications/TPP/

ISBN 1 86134 056 7

The research was funded by the Economic and Social Research Council
(Grant No L311253025) as part of the Local Governance Programme.
Thanks are due to all our respondents, the British Council of Organisations
of Disabled People, the UK Advocacy Network and MINDLINK.

Cover design by Qube Design Associates, Bristol.
Photograph used on front cover supplied by kind permission of Mark
Simmons, Studio BS6 Photography, Bristol.
Printed in Great Britain by Hobbs the Printers Ltd, Southampton.

Contents

1 The policy context   1

2 The research   9

3 Advocacy and joint working: a mental health case study   17

4 Implementing the social model of disability – after the
  honeymoon   47

5 Consumers and citizens   81

6 Conclusion   103

References   111

ONE

The policy context

Introduction

The study reported here concerns the constitution and activity of what we refer to as 'user groups' in the fields of state provision of services for people with mental health problems and with physical disabilities. Although one purpose is to report in some detail on one example of a group operating in each of these fields (in Chapters 3 and 4 respectively), our conclusions also draw on evidence from our research into four other groups (Barnes et al, 1996), and a second purpose is to offer a more general analysis of the relationship of this kind of group to present and future policy options. In this chapter, we outline the context for the report. This can conveniently be divided into two elements, each the subject of a section below: the larger macro-social context *for* policy and the narrower context provided by policy itself, though it is not suggested that these are theoretically or causally unrelated. A third section of this chapter introduces the elements of the 'user movement'.

The context for policy

Much of the thrust of our analysis hinges upon some concept of *citizenship*, a concept which is far from static. Historically, it has been conceived as carrying a complex cluster of meanings: defined legal or social status; means of signifying political identity; a focus of loyalty; a requirement to perform duties; expectations of rights; and a yardstick of good social behaviour (Heater, 1990, p 163). At different historical moments particular elements of this cluster have been emphasised. Thus, for much of the present century until, say, 1980, citizenship has been predominantly discussed from a liberal perspective, that is as a set of *rights* that enables the individual to "function relatively equally in private life or in exchange in civil society" (Meehan, 1993, p 177). T. H. Marshall's (1950) influential analysis of the development over time of, respectively, civil, political and social rights, all counterposed against social class, is the classic text of this genre, which remains at the heart of recent, more sophisticated, sociological accounts such as those of Twine (1994) and Roche (1992).

Over the last two decades, however, the emphasis of discussion has changed in several ways, not all of which are consistent with each other. One shift is the reappearance of the more active 'republican' perspective, that citizenship entails not only rights but a moral duty to "take part in constructing and maintaining [the] community" (Meehan, 1993, p 177; see also Prior et al, 1995). It seems likely that this new emphasis is a response to what is perceived as governmental 'overload': that citizen demands for new public programmes and expenditures are not matched by those for the elimination of old ones (Alford and Friedland, 1985, p 157). It is easy to see the interest of the 'new right' in this shift of emphasis towards the active citizen; it can be used to underpin exhortations for voluntary effort and self-help, and provides a language with which to label policies that de-emphasise the role of the state: 'community care', for instance (Raadschelders, 1995, p 622).

Indeed, this de-emphasis can be taken so far as virtually to dissolve the distinction between citizen and consumer. As Tudor Hart caustically observed on the relationship between neoliberal economics and neoconservative politics assumed by the Conservative governments of the early 1990s:

> **Consumer decisions in the market must always prove wiser, in the long run, than decisions by politicians the consumers elect. Leaders may think they know better, but in the end the best choice is whatever is most profitable, because it suits most consumers in the market. The solution to all social problems is fully to expose them to market forces. Since, in the Conservative view, society and the market are more or less interchangeable terms (anyone not in the market is outside society) market decisions must be democratic because they maximise involvement of consumers; everyone has to buy, but each year fewer people bother to vote. Any attempt to limit the natural behaviour of the market must, therefore, be an infringement of freedom and democracy... (Tudor Hart, 1994, p 66)**

But this logic is not just the result of right-wing political hegemony; there is a sense in which 'republican' exhortations for citizenship as involvement and participation are confronted by an opposing social trend. The 'postmodern' pluralisation of societies into what have been termed 'neotribes' militates against authentic political discourse on anything other than the narrowest self-interest:

> **Most of what passes for public conversation is not that at all. It degenerated as communication lost the check on authenticity provided by dialogue. Outrageous claims ... stand unchallenged, because the media of discourse are monologic.... The macroculture – which is nationwide and crosses generational, class, race, linguistic and gender divisions – [therefore] thins. Thicker, more robust, communities of discourse do develop, but only in enclaves or subcultures, a tendency referred to as neotribalism. (Fox and Miller, 1995, p 7)**

One possible response from welfare state institutions to such social changes is the substitution of vouchers or cash benefits for services: to allow, as it were, consumer choice to arise from citizenship. As we note in Chapter 4, this was popular in the field of physical disability and has been conceded in the form of legislation to enable direct payments to purchase services. The other possible response to these social changes is to seek to rebuild democracy and citizenship through accepting and promoting direct participation of 'neotribes', whose relatively narrow range of interests might allow authentic dialogue about the content and character of welfare state services. The activities of user groups as reported in this study can obviously be seen as attempts to establish just such a dialogue.

Thus, the normative position that citizens ought to play an active part in constructing the community is consistent with several alternative sorts of role for the citizen, none of which are distinctively associated with the political right. They include at least the following:

- a widening of the scope of representative democracy so as to diminish the role of quangos and the 'new magistracy' (Stewart, 1992);
- involvement in user or pressure groups, which in some cases may extend to being seen as new social movements (Dalton and Kuechler, 1990) in order to press for extensions of rights (Knox and McAlister, 1995);
- the provision, sometimes by groups which are also pressure groups, sometimes financed by the state, sometimes financed charitably, of services either as an alternative to those provided by the state, or in the absence of state provision;

• the incorporation of the citizen into the process of decision making about the extent or character of state provision, through such devices as 'citizens' juries' (Cooper et al, 1995; Coote and Lenaghan, 1997).

This multiplicity of approaches both reflects and responds to the debates and macro-social change outlined above and leads directly to a consideration of the public policy against the background of which our study was conducted. The normative requirement for greater democracy is confronted by increased difficulty in delivering it. Rhodes (1997) has noted that the pluralisation described above has also come to characterise the field of public policy in the UK, which is increasingly governed by *networks* of public and private institutions operating in their own interests. Thus the core State has been 'hollowed out' along several dimensions: upwards (as a result of European institutions); laterally (as a result of the creation of 'agencies' to deliver public services and the massive expansion of 'quangos' run by government appointees); and downwards (as a result of increasing privatisation). In consequence, the State is increasingly unable to control policy and private government has been substituted for public government, or 'governance' for government.

User involvement: the policy background

The idea that public services should be more responsive to their users is a standard element in the doctrine of the 'new public management' (Pollitt, 1993). User involvement is now treated as a policy imperative for the National Health Service (NHS) as a whole, but it has a rather longer history in respect of certain parts of the service than of others. In particular, the therapeutic models (such as 'normalisation'; Wolfensberger, 1972) which underpinned care of what were then referred to as mentally handicapped people placed great emphasis upon the rights of clients and patients to exercise independence over their current and future lifestyles, including in respect of the treatment and care that they received. Such involvement was seen not only as having an instrumental (therapeutic) value but as being intrinsically valuable as an ordinary human right:

> **Mentally handicapped people have the same human value as anyone else and also the same human rights. Living in the community is both a right and a need. Services must recognise the individuality of mentally handicapped people. (King's Fund, 1980, p14)**

These assumptions were incorporated into a number of localised initiatives and experiments developed from within local authorities and health services (Towell, 1988; Barnes and Wistow, 1991; 1994) and ostensibly found official favour in the more general policy of 'community care' as it developed in the 1980s and early 1990s. Thus, the White Paper *Caring for people* (Secretaries of State, 1989, para 1.8) stated that its proposals for what has subsequently been referred to as the 'purchaser/provider split' in community care were intended to "give people a greater individual say in how they live their lives and the services they need to help them do so". User inputs were to be made at both meso and micro levels of the system; each local authority was required to consult a wide range of stakeholders, including representatives of users and of the general public, as well as to ensure that individuals' needs assessments took account of their, and their carers', wishes (Wistow and Hardy, 1994). Research focusing on user input to needs assessment and community care planning demonstrated just how difficult many professionals found it to engage in genuine and open dialogue with service users at both individual and collective levels (Ellis, 1993; Lindow and Morris, 1994).

The introduction to the UK welfare state of the purchaser/provider split in 1991 was not confined to community care, but extended to all health care. A central element in such organisational arrangements was the weakening of the influence of provider vested interests (Harrison, 1991) in order to allow health authorities (HAs) to "concentrate on and listen to the user without the pressure to favour their own service provision" (Audit Commission, 1992, para 20). Although appointed rather than elected, such authorities were officially represented as 'champions of the people', purchasing on behalf of their local residents and in response to needs and priorities identified by 'local voices' (NHS Management Executive, 1992). One of the Department of Health's six medium-term priorities was that HAs should

> ... **give greater voice and emphasis to users of NHS services and their carers in their own care, the development and definition of standards set for NHS services locally and the development of NHS policy both locally and nationally. (NHS Executive, 1995, p 9)**

The mechanisms which should be used for such purposes were not centrally specified and HAs were left to make local decisions to employ a number of the approaches listed in the preceding section, including ad hoc surveys of the public and of large employers, standing public panels of questionnaire respondents, and various face-to-face approaches such as focus groups and citizens' juries (Dowswell et al, 1997).

The field work which we report in later chapters was conducted before the general election of May 1997, since which a number of further policy changes have been introduced. One of these involves the direct collection of user opinion: there is to be an annual national survey of patient and user opinion (Secretary of State for Health, 1997 p 65). Another involves the inclusion of user representatives on the national groups which will steer the production of 'National Service Frameworks', that is evidence-based models of clinical service delivery to which NHS service providers will be expected to adhere (NHS Executive, 1998, p 27). One of the first of these will relate to mental health services. Health care consumers are also formally involved in shaping the NHS Research and Development Programme through the Standing Advisory Group on Consumer Involvement.

User groups

Not surprisingly, neither these official approaches to user involvement nor their semi-official predecessors have always satisfied users, though they did provide some legitimation for the activities of those who sought to develop their own organisations and activities 'bottom up'. The British Council of Organisations of Disabled People was formed in 1981 in response to dissatisfaction both with statutory services and with the control of voluntary organisations by able-bodied people. 'People First', an organisation founded in the USA to promote self-advocacy by people with learning difficulties, was established in the UK in 1984 (Williams and Schoultz, 1984), a time which also saw the foundation of the first mental health Patients' Councils on a model developed in the Netherlands (Gell, 1987). These and groups formed more recently can be seen as part of a growing 'user movement' with links throughout Europe (van der Male, 1995) and the USA.

The kinds of group which were the subject of our study are variously categorised by their membership and by those whom they seek to influence. 'Self-help groups', 'pressure groups', 'consumer groups' and 'advocacy groups' are all current terms. The term 'user' (and hence 'user group') is not unproblematic. First, many physically disabled people do not give priority to services in the usual sense of personal services of the kind provided by (for instance) health and social care professionals; their emphasis, based upon a social model of disability (see Chapter 4) is more upon desired modifications of the physical and social environment. Second, in certain contexts 'user' can carry the pejorative connotations of drug abuse. Third, some groups and individuals prefer to describe themselves in other terms; 'survivors' is the preferred term of members of the organisation of mental health service users, 'Survivors Speak Out'. Finally, it may be objected that the term 'user' imparts a kind of false neutrality to the subject, implying that the individual's status as a service user is unproblematic, whereas in fact it may be the result of professional 'labelling' and (in the mental health field) be entirely involuntary. Nevertheless, a shorthand label for the subject of our study is necessary, and the objections to 'user groups' seemed not to be overwhelming.

The feature that distinguishes the kind of groups in our study from the mass of interest groups operating in the field is that they are *self-organised* by the recipients of services and those affected by official policy in the relevant sector (mental health or physical disability). The detailed constitutions and objectives of our exemplar groups are set out in Chapters 3 and 4, but in general terms the objectives of user groups concern greater autonomy for their members and other users of the same services. Some such claims to autonomy relate to the content and quality of statutory services and are therefore made against the managers and professionals who run and provide such services; we discuss the response of such 'officials' to these claims in Chapters 3 and 4. However, other autonomy claims, such as those concerning social exclusion, are much broader than can be delivered by officials within the context of welfare state institutions as presently constituted. All the groups that we studied were concerned with either mental health or physical disabilities, fields in which both social care and health care are important. However, there are many other user groups in other fields to whom this also applies, groups representing people with HIV/AIDS, for instance. What is at present less clear (though see Wood, forthcoming) is how far groups operating in sectors closer to acute medicine are also making autonomy claims which go beyond the specific content of services.

TWO

The research

Introduction

As noted in Chapter 1, users of health and social care services have become increasingly organised, and within this, increasingly *self-organised*. Although there are signs that this process is spreading to other sectors of care, including acute medicine, it is in the fields of mental health problems, learning difficulties and physical disability that it has been most long-standing; these are the roots of the user movement. We sought to take advantage of this relative maturity as a means to understanding the implications of user self-organisation for developing concepts of citizenship. The research was therefore confined to these sectors, and a comparison of mental health and physical disability was chosen as one which provided a potentially useful contrast between a sector largely concerned with personal services (mental health) and one with a much wider focus, including services but also the environment and the social origins of 'disability'. We did not, however, start out by identifying particular user groups for study: we describe below how they were identified.

Research objectives

Our research objectives were both policy-related and conceptual; the former centred on the relationship of user group activity to new forms of agency management, and the latter on notions of consumerism and citizenship as a means of understanding the significance of user groups. The separate perspectives of user groups and actors within the statutory agencies (whom we term 'officials') were also to be addressed. In summary, our objectives were to use a purposive sample of user groups in each of the two specified service sectors to analyse

- (from the perspective of the user groups) the topics on which influence was sought, the strategies employed, and their resulting influence within the system of local governance;
- (from the perspective of officials) the legitimacy accorded to groups

and their specific activities, the strategies adopted for dealing with them, and the place accorded to them within the wider context of official activity.

Overall, our objectives were to examine this activity in the context of contemporary notions of consumerism and citizenship.

Selecting the user groups

The research adopted a case study design. Our starting point was user self-organisation rather than official 'user involvement' strategies. As intended, we studied three mental health groups and three disabled people's groups. Following meetings with national umbrella organisations, local groups were selected to enable exploration of different strategies for achieving influence. Users of services have objected to being subjected to the professional gaze of researchers as they are also objecting to being constructed as passive recipients of welfare services. In some instances they have refused to participate in research projects. We were advised that some groups would be likely to reject an approach from us. In each case we discussed the nature of the research with the groups we approached and agreed with them the way in which we would select and approach interviewees, and feed back results. Considerable discussion was required before one particular group finally agreed to be involved. The groups eventually selected were as follows.

Mental health user groups

Group One, established in 1986, is an umbrella organisation supporting user councils and advocacy projects throughout the city. Membership, approximately 60 at the time of the research, is not a prerequisite for participation and is open to users and others committed to its aims. The group aims to influence service provision both locally and nationally. Its tactics emphasise partnership rather than campaigning. It has been funded by local and health authorities and charitable donations. Interviewees described it as a 'broad church' in representing the individual and collective voices of users. It is located in territory covered by a county council and city council (both Labour controlled) in the process of becoming a unitary authority.

Group Two is a small campaigning group of users and ex-users working within the local MIND organisations. There is no membership, but communication with users is maintained through an advice and information line and through campaigning. The group participates in health service planning. It runs advocacy projects funded by health authorities within hospital and primary care services. The group has a poor relationship with one local social services department, but works more effectively with another. Campaigning is not funded although the group has income from property rentals. It is located in a Labour controlled metropolitan district.

Group Three is a democratically run drop-in service, aimed at younger people with mental health problems. It acts as a support and self-help group. Part of the group's building is designated as women's space. Within this largely unstructured environment activities can be organised according to the interests of users. The group is reluctant to become involved with officials and rarely campaigns. It is funded through charities and by grants from statutory agencies. It is located in a Labour controlled metropolitan district.

Disabled people's groups

Group Four, established in 1992, was initiated by a jointly funded development officer to facilitate consultation with disabled people. The group has a role in the statutory service planning process. It does not yet have a constitution. Interviewees were uncertain about what type of group they consider themselves to be: a support group or a pressure group. They do not have independent funding. Membership is approximately 50. It is located in a Conservative controlled metropolitan district.

Group Five is a well-established coalition of disabled people founded in 1981. It was one of the first in the country and has a strong influence both locally and nationally. It is a representative democracy asserting the right of disabled people to be fully participating citizens. Members are committed to the social model of disability. It is a campaigning and pressure group. Only disabled people can vote and hold office but able-bodied people can become associate members. Membership has fluctuated between 300 and 900. The group has a provider arm through which it works in partnership with the statutory agencies. It is also involved in planning and consultative forums. It receives funding from the county council and a district council and has in the past received joint funding. It is located in territory covered by Labour controlled county and city councils (in the process of becoming a unitary authority), and a Labour controlled district council.

Group Six was established in 1981 under the auspices of the local Council for Voluntary Service. It aims to represent disabled people and has an established consultative role. It provides advice and information and carries out campaigns. There is no formal membership. Disabled people act as volunteers on the advice and information service and as representatives within the consultative process. Funding comes from the city council, local social services and the health authority. The group adopted a constitution after the research period. At the time of our interviews a separate action group provided more of a campaigning arm. The group is located in territory covered by a 'hung' county council and Labour controlled city council in the process of becoming a unitary authority.

In this report, we examine the activities of and responses to groups One (Chapter 3) and Five (Chapter 4) in greater detail than has been possible in other publications arising from the project. (See References for other publications.)

Identifying interviewees

User respondents in each group were identified through discussion with initial contacts. All were 'activists', although we aimed to include people occupying different positions within the groups. After these respondents had been interviewed, we identified 'official' respondents from the user group studies. User transcripts were scrutinised for names or job titles of respondents. This was augmented by the use of snowballing techniques. Officials who had had contact with groups and who were the recipients of 'influence' were interviewed to explore their reactions to this and to the groups more generally. We included managers, professionals and politicians among official respondents. The official respondents worked in social and health services (on both sides of the purchaser/provider split), and in other local authority departments. Politicians included local councillors and MPs.

The official respondents do not comprise 'groups' in the way that the user respondents do. If our starting point had been official strategies for user involvement the interviewees may have been different. The time factor was also significant. The majority of the user groups had been active since the early to mid-1980s. Some of the officials identified in interviews were no longer working in the area. At a time of major reorganisation in (especially NHS) services the rapid turnover of staff meant that many of the officials were reflecting on a much shorter period than user respondents had done.

We interviewed 46 users and 66 officials, including one telephone interview, and collected extensive documentary evidence, including press cuttings. Interviews were tape-recorded and transcribed, and analysed for their thematic content using 'The Ethnograph' software. The characteristics of the user and official respondents are set out in Tables 1 and 2 respectively (pp 15-16).

Impact of the research on user groups

Researchers working in this area have had to develop new ways of working with users as participants rather than subjects of the research process. Our project was neither user led, nor truly participative. There were a number of reasons for this, not least because our interest was in exploring the perspectives of officials as well as the views of users themselves. Nevertheless, we sought to adopt an open approach to the research to enable users to be 'active subjects' rather than simply 'respondents'. User motivation for involvement in the groups derived from negative experiences of services, or from the effects of stigma and discrimination. This was seen to give people the legitimacy to seek change in services and the professional definition of their 'problems', and to work for justice and fair treatment more generally. Interviewees also believed they had something to offer people in similar situations. Shared histories and identities were important in creating an environment supportive of collective action. Participation within the group was experienced as valuable in its own right and encouraged people to remain active. As we will see, some groups include research as one of their own strategies for achieving change. Motivation to be involved in our project was in part a sense that this might provide another route for their voices to be heard. But agreement to participate was dependent on our preparedness to be open and responsive to the different ways in which each group operated. For some this meant attending meetings of group representatives to explain the research and be questioned on it, in other cases contact was made with key individuals who then introduced our proposals to group members themselves.

We produced individual case study reports for each group and obtained responses to these before finalising them. At the completion of fieldwork we held a feedback meeting for representatives from the user groups studied. Four of the groups attended and welcomed the opportunity to meet together. In the meeting, users indicated that the distinction between consumerist and citizenship approaches was a useful analysis which would help them review their objectives and strategies. One group talked of having learned the language of consumerism, but of not being completely happy with this. This group subsequently invited one of us to speak at an event they were organising on behalf of the regional NHS Executive in order to emphasise the significance of a 'citizenship' perspective on disabled people's experiences. Users wanted to know whether officials viewed them as citizens and talked of ways in which citizenship could be constrained by administrative action. Hopes that contact would be maintained were expressed. Involvement in the research appeared to be particularly significant for the 'newest' group which was not linked into the broader disabled people's movement. One group intended to use the material in negotiations with officials. It was suggested that our findings would be valuable to other user groups and represented an important reflection on the current and future nature of the welfare state.

However, interviewees in one group had found it uncomfortable to have their words reflected back to them in the case study report. They were concerned that other group members would be able to recognise who had said what, even though individuals had not been identified. This concern perhaps reflected two things: first, that expectations about 'research' may be shaped by quantitative research methods and thus the quite detailed textual analysis we undertook came as a surprise; and second, that members of this group may have been less used to debating with each other some of the issues we were raising with them. Our report may have documented differences of perspective which had not yet been addressed internally. This response was an important reminder of the way in which 'scrutiny' by researchers – even when the approach is intended to be open and negotiated – can create unintended difficulties.

Table 1: The groups

	Mental health or disability	Date established	Type of organisation	Constitution	Funding	Membership	Relationship with service providers/ purchasers	Other activities
Group One	Mental health	1986	Umbrella partnership group	Democratic	Health authority, local authority, charity	Approx 60, anyone supporting aims can join	Influence at local and national level	Advocacy, advice and information
Group Two	Mental health		Small campaigning group	Under local MIND organisation	Health authority, rent from property	No membership	Involved with NHS planning, poor relationship with social services	Advice and info service, advocacy project
Group Three	Mental health	1986/87	User run drop-in for younger people with mental health problems	Democratic	Social services, health authority, charity	Very flexible, fluctuating members	Do not seek to establish relationship	Social activities, some individual campaigning & advocacy, women's space
Group Four	Disability	1992	Support/self-help/pressure group	No constitution	None. Funding available from development officer (joint finance)	Approx 50, disabled people only	Role in service planning. Group originally established by service providers	
Group Five	Disability	1981	Coalition, campaigning and pressure group	Representative democracy	Local authority. Previously joint funding	Fluctuated between 300 and 900, anyone can join, only disabled people vote	Strong influence locally/ nationally	Involvement in centre for integrated living
Group Six	Disability	1981/82	1. Umbrella organisation with 2. Smaller campaigning and pressure group within it	Under local CVS organisation	1. County council, health authority 2. No direct funding	1. None, users act as representatives in consultation process 2. 20-30 members, only disabled people	1. Established consultation role 2. Less developed consultation role	Advice and info, some advocacy

Table 2: Official respondents

	Nature of authority	Local authority		National Health Service		Professional	Politicians/other
		Social services	Other	Purchaser	Provider		
Group One mental health	County council (Labour controlled), City council (Labour) becoming unitary authority	Head of Partnership, Head of Health and Disability Policy, Principal Mental Health Officer, Head ASW Training		Quality Assurance Officers	Quality Advisor, Rehabilitation and Community Care Managers, Medical Director	Consultant Psychiatrists	Director of Council for Voluntary Service
Group Two mental health	City council (Labour), metropolitan district	Mental Health Resources Manager, Assistant Director		Commissioning Manager, Senior Policy Advisor	Development Officer, Clinical Audit	Consultant Psychiatrists	
Group Three mental health	City council (Labour), metropolitan	Planning Officer		Director of Strategic & Corporate Development	Deputy Director of Mental Health Services, User Involvement Facilitator	Clinical Psychologist	
Group Four disability	Metropolitan borough council (Conservative controlled)	Assistant Director, two joint funded posts with NHS provider	Road Safety Officer, Head of Building Control	Director of Health Commissioning	General Manager Specialist Services Development Officer, Manager Wheelchair Services		Chairperson Social Services Committee, Councillor, Chief Exec Special Needs Bus Company
Group Five disability	County council (Labour), City council (Labour) becoming unitary authority, district council (Labour)	Planning Officers, Development Officer, Area Manager	Personnel Officer	Principal Assistant Director of Planning & Information, Director of Community Affairs	Rehabilitation Services Manager	National Park Landscape Architect	District Council Leader, County Councillors, Local MP, CHC Officer, Voluntary Sector Provider
Group Six disability	County council (hung Conservative/Liberal Democrat), City council (Labour) becoming unitary authority	Head of Adult Services, Principal Officer Planning and Commissioning	Disablement Officer, Economic Development Officer, Head of Housing Needs, Head of Building Control, Personnel Officer	Corporate Planner Community Care	Deputy Chief Executive		City Councillor, Chairperson Disabled Advisory Group, Local MP

THREE

Advocacy and joint working: a mental health case study

In this chapter we discuss the way in which a well-established group of mental health service users is working to ensure that users are influential within local service systems and more widely. We start by reporting on the way in which activists describe the nature of the group, its objectives and ways of working, and then go on to consider how 'officials' in local health and social care agencies are responding to them.

Mental health service users have been organising themselves in this particular city since the mid-1980s. The city-wide organisation had its origins in user councils on hospital wards and developed in the first instance as a Patients' Councils Support Group. The development was thus a 'bottom-up' initiative, firmly located in the day-to-day experiences of current service users who wanted to achieve more influence over the services they were receiving, and to play their part in service planning. The following description refers to the period 1994-95 when data were collected.

Constitution, structure and funding

The city-wide group is a company limited by guarantee, and a registered charity. It employs three part-time and two full-time paid workers – discriminating in favour of people who are or have been users of services. There are also 20-25 regular volunteers, mainly users, who often work practically full-time. The management committee has 15 members, at least half of whom have to be users, and is elected by the membership. Paid workers do not have voting rights on the management committee, but do attend meetings.

Mental health services in the city are organised into six sectors and the group has a representative in each of these sectors. The volunteers attend meetings in their sector, canvass opinion and report back to the 'Interlink' meeting, where representatives from the different sectors meet together monthly.

In addition to the sector groups there are resident-only meetings on wards and client-only meetings in day hospitals and day centres. These are supported by workers and volunteers and they receive administrative and organisational back up. All groups are represented on the city Patients' User Council which also includes among its membership representatives from the Joint Specialist Planning Team, the local Trust; a link worker from one of the sector teams; the Relatives' Support Group; users from the rehabilitation services; black and Asian groups; and the Chair of the city Patients' Council Support Group. In addition, managers, planners and professionals are invited to Council meetings to discuss particular issues of relevance to them.

A separate initiative supported by the group (Ecoworks) provides employment training and rehabilitation through involvement in ecological work projects.

Funding

Funding comes from a variety of sources. At the time of the research:
- The **district health authority** provided funding for two posts, office rent, volunteer expenses, and a part-time administrative worker.
- Mainstream **social services** funding paid for the worker supporting the Citizen Advocacy Scheme, while funding from the Service Standards Inspection Unit (SSD) paid for a one-year research project. The Mental Health Development Budget provided approximately £500 each for user groups.
- The **Mental Health NHS Trust** provided £380 for volunteers' expenses.
- **The Mental Health Foundation, plus joint finance, plus a local brewery** paid for the Patient Advocacy Scheme worker for two years.
- A worker appointed to develop initiatives in the rehabilitation services was funded for three years by **joint finance.**
- Ad hoc funding for specific projects had been received from local private firms as well as from health and social services agencies.

Much of this funding is time limited. Inadequate or insecure funding is a source of concern for group members. It makes volunteer recruitment difficult as well as meaning insecure futures for both projects and project workers.

Membership

Membership is free and open to anyone living in the area who supports the objectives of the group, who makes an application to join and who is elected by the Management Committee. Members are not required to adhere to a set of beliefs or aims, other than a commitment to the right of service users to have their voices heard.

The majority of active members are users or ex-users of mental health services, but membership is not restricted to users. At the time the interviews were conducted the group had approximately 60 individual members, including two consultant psychiatrists. Because of its umbrella group structure, individual membership per se is not considered a priority. Building contacts and ensuring people know about and can access the group is seen as more important than recruiting individual members. Advocacy on behalf of both members and non-members is considered more important in maintaining contact with service users and identifying issues for action, than is member attendance at management committee meetings or the AGM.

However, several interviewees noted that many people with a mental health problem do not have any contact with the group and that there continues to be a need to find ways of giving them a voice. They recognised that credibility is related to the breadth and depth of involvement within the group and they are concerned to maximise their contact with users in different circumstances. In particular there are some categories of user groups who are not considered to be well represented within the group.

A majority of interviewees saw lack of involvement from black, Asian and other minority ethnic group users as a significant limitation. Activists were not sure how to tackle this issue. Meetings have been held with black and Asian groups but because the group is seen as white-dominated, black users are reluctant to attend. Black groups always receive minutes and invitations to attend meetings. Two interviewees thought the group should not try to involve black and Asian groups or individuals directly but rather that they should support the existing black and Asian groups by passing on useful information.

One respondent also talked of the need to attract younger members. The average age of members is creeping up and this was reflected in the ages of those we interviewed, only one of whom was under 40.

One interviewee highlighted the lack of active involvement of people with the most disabling mental health problems, and those who are only seen sporadically, for example by a Community Psychiatric Nurse or by their GP. Once users have left hospital it is difficult to maintain contact as information about discharged patients is confidential and can only be shared with their agreement.

Nevertheless, workers from the group are involved with a wide range of settings and attempt to involve many different users in the various forums in which they engage in discussions with officials. They encourage users to take on active roles when they are ready for this. They believe that they have achieved credibility with purchasers, providers and service users, although they are continually looking for ways to ensure that they are able to include and represent the experiences of as many mental health service users as possible.

Achieving influence

Our discussion in Chapter 1 of changes within the health and social care system demonstrated the way in which user involvement has come to be legitimated as a policy objective. This group, in common with many others, came into existence before user involvement became accepted as a responsibility of health and social care agencies, and before community care changes were consolidated by the 1990 NHS and Community Care Act. Those who have been active in the group from the start had experienced, and indeed contributed to, substantial policy shifts at both local and national level. Like those involved in the disabled people's coalition described in Chapter 4, some of those we interviewed were able to reflect on changing relationships between users and officials, as well as on the broader policy changes within which these relationships were being negotiated. Some had longer experience of service delivery and policy making than the officials with whom they were working.

There was concern among group members about the shortage of money available to resource health and social care services. They saw the potential benefits of community care policy being compromised by under-resourcing. One felt that the group should be seeking to influence the overall level of funding as well as the way in which services were being provided. One interviewee expressed disappointment that there was no sign of legislation to make community care services entitlements, while others were not convinced that the large institutions had disappeared for good and felt that psychiatric hospitals would always be needed. But regardless of the way in which the nature of service provision might change, interviewees saw a continuing role for the group in representing those receiving mental health services, whether that be in hospital or community settings.

While those who had been active for some time acknowledged the higher profile achieved by user involvement, there was also a sense that the full significance of this had not been grasped by officials:

> **"... because they have this policy of user involvement even though some of them don't know what they are getting themselves into."**

In this context, the group had established a coherent role and identity as an advocacy group prepared to work with officials, but also prepared to oppose and challenge as necessary.

Objectives, activities and influence

The broad aims of the group are "to promote the interests of the users and ex-users of the psychiatric services in (town)" (Memorandum of Association). These aims are achieved through the provision of advice, assistance, education and information, as well as through promoting the participation of users and ex-users in the management of services.

There are three core elements to the activities supported by the group:

- **Self-advocacy:** this is mainly achieved through the various user groups, including Patients' Councils and community-based groups. It is primarily concerned with the development of individual empowerment and influence through collective means.
- **Patient advocacy:** "Concentrating on Individual Advocacy for people who need more one-to-one advice when dealing with their concerns" (from project description).
- **Citizen advocacy:** finding advocates for people who are least able to exert influence on their own behalf.

The group has a contract with the health authority to make a specified number of advocacy contacts a year.

Advocacy services have developed in different service settings from their origins in work with hospital in-patients. For example, at the time of the research a project based in residential homes was underway. In each context, the group seeks to create ways in which users of mental health services can influence current and future services. Which issues are prioritised for action is largely determined by the individuals or groups concerned, although workers may also suggest topics worthy of consideration. One example of an issue introduced by group workers for consideration was the use of forms to enable users to undertake their own assessment of their needs. The purpose in such instances is to raise awareness of possibilities, rather than to impose an agenda.

In addition to advocacy, the group is represented on joint planning committees and other working groups, and also undertakes education and training of mental health workers.

The group also has aims which relate to people's lives beyond their role as service users or 'consumers'. All interviewees agreed that improving employment opportunities, improving access to educational and training opportunities, influencing the public's perception of people with mental health problems and establishing alliances with other groups figured among their aims. Nine out of the ten respondents also thought that the group aimed to improve access to leisure and recreation facilities.

Broader political and cultural objectives were also identified. Nine people said that the group aimed to increase participation in local and/ or national politics and also to change the way in which people with mental health problems are portrayed in the media. Achieving rights to specified services was identified as an objective by eight members of the group, while six people saw both achieving anti-discrimination legislation and achieving amendments to existing welfare legislation as group objectives.

The thinking underpinning the ecological work projects makes links between environmentalism and the creation of lifestyles which are protective of people's mental health (Davey, 1994; 1999). The activist who has taken the lead on these developments expressed his underlying philosophy as follows:

> **"I've felt for a very long time that mental health and mental health issues are either about the fundamental problems of human existence which everybody relates to, or it's a very narrow specialism within medicine understood by only a few neurologists, and I incline to the former view. And I think that widening out the ideas so that people can see their mental health as being about their emotional life, about their relationships, about their relationship to the environment and so on, and seeing so-called mental health problems as symptoms, or mental illness symptoms as being extreme versions of what everybody experiences – it seems to me is the way to break down stigma which people with mental health problems face. It's an aspect of re-integration of people with mental health problems and it's a different way of seeing re-evaluation of the quality of life which is very important**

for the Green movement and all sorts of political, social processes."

While this perspective is being developed outside the group's mainstream action in advocacy and participation in service planning, it is consistent with the group's broader objectives of breaking down stigma and supporting the participation of people with mental health problems in a wide range of social activities. It reflects an analysis of the experience of 'mental illness' which challenges medical models in a similar way to the challenge offered by the social model of disability. While the group's overall objectives are not located within this analysis in the way in which the disabled people's coalition located objectives within the social model of disability, it continues to provide a basis for alternative models of 'services' which are being developed under the group's umbrella. The significance of such models may increase as both public health and environmental issues achieve a higher profile, and as the importance of linking the health and regeneration agendas is being recognised in the context of Health Action Zones and other initiatives based in public health models.

Methods and tactics

As we have suggested, the group adopts a number of different methods in order to pursue its objectives.

Partnership or joint working

In our discussions with national user network representatives when we were defining research questions, there was some hesitation about the concept of 'partnership' between user organisations and statutory agencies because of the unequal power relationships involved. We have used the term 'joint working' instead to indicate circumstances in which users are participants in joint enterprises, but without making any assumptions about the power relationships within those enterprises.

Members of the group were engaged in action and seeking change at different levels within the mental health system. At national level, a member of the group was involved in the Mental Health Task Force User Group set up to provide user input to the development and implementation of community care policy.

At the local level there are a number of forums in which the group makes an input to strategic decision making. These are the city-wide meetings with mental health unit managers and others in the Patients' Council; 'Interlink', which is a collective forum in which representatives from the sector groups come together; and meetings with the (then) district health authority to influence the content of contracts. Through Ecoworks there are also strategic links with local district councils and the county council.

Also at strategic level the closure of the long-stay hospital provided an opportunity for the group to play a part in determining the future pattern of services. While input to service planning was seen as a priority, some interviewees were reluctant to become involved in decision making about resource allocation and prioritisation because this would mean that they could be associated with decisions to cut services. Other responses suggested that the role of the group was to call decision makers to account for such decisions, rather than to be part of the decision-making process itself. Thus, rather than having isolated users attend board meetings, health service managers were being called to account by the Patients' Council:

> **"I think the Patients' Council works well because it does work on the principle that it's not one or two service users … sitting on the edge of a meeting or a trust board or a management meeting or whatever, it is managers, senior managers coming to meetings of service users to be accountable and really they have to account on the spot."**

At the time of interviews the potential for involvement in contract specification as a means of achieving strategic influence was still being explored. There was some feeling that the group was taking more responsibility for identifying failures to meet the terms of contracts than were the purchasers. While this, too, was seen to be a way of calling providers to account, group members were reluctant to let purchasers off the hook by undertaking what they rightly saw to be the monitoring role of purchasers.

While respondents thought it was important that the group should continue to develop influence over strategic issues, there was also a commitment to pursue service-specific issues of immediate concern to users:

> **"It's still vitally important that folks have a say about what is happening to them on a ward or a day centre, or whatever,**

you know, because to them at that particular time that's important."

One of the group's strengths is the way in which its structure enables it to operate at all levels and to make links between them. Issues arising at an individual level are picked up through individual advocacy and these can also be taken up at service level or at strategic level if appropriate. Thus when the mental health unit said that it could not afford to prescribe Clozapine to particular patients, the group not only took this up with providers on behalf of the individuals concerned, but also took this up with purchasers with the outcome that the purchasers provided money for a trial run.

Research, training and alternative models

The group monitors what users think about services and uses this as a way of identifying issues to take up with providers. One interviewee saw the wider potential of research which had not yet been realised:

"I would like to see — do some more … user-led research and research linked to … general alternatives and ideas of different therapies and things, which is happening to some extent already, but we also research much more on some of the theoretical things like types of legislation we want to see …"

If its role in research was as yet undeveloped, the group had significant input into training mental health professionals and managers. Training was seen as a practical way of trying to achieve new understandings of people's distress. One person described an awareness-raising workshop for nurses led by members. She thought this was an effective way of changing attitudes – "if you get them young enough!" Group members are also involved in induction training for all staff – from cleaners to psychiatrists to managers; in social work qualifying training; and in courses for Approved Social Workers (ASWs) in the county and neighbouring authorities.

The importance of influencing attitudes and understandings is seen to be a much wider task than that of training mental health workers. For the previous two years the group had held a Mental Health Awareness Week. This has continued as an annual event aiming to influence public perceptions and understandings of mental distress. One method used is a 'Stress Game' designed to make the link between mental health problems and the stresses which everyone experiences as part of ordinary life: poverty, relationships, bereavement, for example.

As we described above, the group's involvement in ecological work projects has been developed on the basis of an analysis of the experience of mental disorder which substantially rejects medical models of mental illness. Not all those we interviewed rejected a medical model, but most spoke of a wish to challenge professional definitions of people's problems and of the need to develop alternative interventions, such as aromatherapy.

Delivering alternatives?

Activists do not see the group as significantly involved in providing services which might be considered to offer alternatives to statutory mental health services. They do aim to ensure alternative forms of treatment are available within mainstream services and to ensure that users have access to information which will enable them to make choices betweeen, for example, medication and 'talking treatments'. They have also used their influence to get an aromatherapy service provided at the acute hospital, and they have obtained money to purchase a caravan which enables people with mental health problems to take affordable holidays. Both emphasise the importance of non-medical interventions and can be considered to represent *additions* to the services available.

A common need identified by users of mental health services is for services which are available outside normal office hours. One of the consultants in the city had suggested that if such a service were to be developed it would be better provided by the group than by the health service. No decision about this had been reached within the research period, but there was considerable uncertainty within the group about taking on a service provider role.

Using the market

The opportunity to become involved in quite detailed contract specification is an example of how the purchaser/provider split introduced a new mechanism through which influence could be exerted. Two examples were given of where the group had influenced contracts: first, the requirement to provide information about services and about medication, and second, the requirement to provide aftercare services following discharge. There was also a view that contracting might provide an opportunity for broadening the range of services available. Discussing the provision of alternative forms of treatment, one person said:

> **"We can actually say, 'Well, can you put it into next year's contract or the next five years' contract or is there an organisation that wants to set themselves up and bid for money from the health authority to do that?'"**

The group is contracted to provide advocacy services, but the contract is neither detailed nor closely monitored. One person discussed the dilemmas that would be associated with the group contracting to provide its own services apart from advocacy:

> **"What I would see is — supporting groups of individuals to set up provision and supporting them to apply for money or to compete for that money, but unless — had another arm that became its providing arm, then I think it would be very difficult and I think the other thing for me is about if we are an advocacy project and we are also providing services, then technically we could be arguing against ourselves if those services aren't appropriate for individuals. So I'm not wholly convinced that being a provider and an advocacy group can go hand in hand."**

At an individual level enabling people to purchase services directly was not seen as a priority. Only one interviewee thought that might be something they would want to pursue.

Campaigning and politics

Campaigning is not seen as a deliberate strategy. However, particular issues may be pursued in ways which might be considered to constitute a 'campaign'. Amending the 'no-smoking' policy in hospital wards was suggested as an example. On more wide-ranging issues it appeared that if the group adopted a deliberate campaigning stance this could be experienced as threatening by officials. One interviewee felt that providers had been very uncomfortable when one of the local user groups supported by the city-wide group had campaigned against plans for service developments in their area. This had included writing letters to local MPs and had produced a reaction which was described as follows:

> **"I think somehow the Trust thought there was a kind of**

internal discipline within — that we would operate in a set way using the available mechanisms..."

Although the city-wide group has developed useful joint working relationships with officials, it will not try to prevent the groups it supports from adopting other methods to achieve their objectives. It has also itself lobbied politicians in relation to anti-discrimination legislation. The importance of support from MPs and others beyond the local mental health services was recognised:

"I think both to secure funding and to go forward, we need to get ourselves in, our ideas in the public arena a lot more and that means to go beyond the mental health services, to me ... we need to get a recognition in broader political circles and that's where I think our safety lies."

Involvement at a national level is one way of achieving recognition beyond the local mental health services and creating an environment in which views of users are more likely to be taken seriously. Involvement in the Mental Health Task Force provided one opportunity for this, as did input to the UK Advocacy Network, Survivors Speak Out and MIND evidence to the Select Committee on the issue of Supervision Orders (an extension of powers to supervise certain people previously detained under the 1983 Mental Health Act).

Relationships with services

At the time of the research the group had been in existence for eight years. During that time the reorganisation of services had resulted in new types of agencies with which relationships had to be established, and introduced new mechanisms around which such relationships had to be negotiated.

Local circumstances had changed. For example, a change in personnel had affected the relationship with social services while reorganisation led to the loss of a specific post with a mental health brief, resulting in a much more tenuous relationship.

"Now the channels of communication into social services are to somebody who's got a multiple responsibility for all disability issues and planning ... so it's a mess from a mental health point of view."

The group itself had developed in confidence as an organisation, as had the individuals within the group. One person commented that when it was first established, "Management and professionals were frightened to death ... horrified to think that there were people who were trying to have a say in our professional treatment".

Eight years on it was considered rare for managers to try to do something without consulting the group. Workers are well known on the wards and ward meetings led by members are well accepted.

The development of the advocacy movement generally has given added confidence and legitimacy to those acting in this role: "I suppose I have more confidence in challenging than I had then because there is now this understanding that it is acceptable to be an advocate".

Gradually contacts between the group and officials have been established higher in the hierarchy. Health service managers are considered to be more prepared to be more accountable to users:

> **"Six years ago, the idea of saying to management we'd like you to come and meet with a group of twenty users to listen to what they think about the services you are providing would have been a joke. Unheard of. But people are used to that now."**

However, not everyone was convinced that this was anything more than a superficial change. One interviewee who had been involved with the group for two years felt the relationship with officials had been largely consistent over that period. It may be that the major shift in thinking about user involvement had taken place in the city by the early 1990s and that any subsequent changes have been marginal.

Comments made by interviewees describe a generally amicable relationship with an ease of communication: "I think there's very open lines in between times to try and pass comments, get things done, set up ad hoc meetings on particular issues if the need arises".

The relationship with the health service was generally considered to be better than that with social services. One interviewee claimed that people from the health authority would turn up to the meetings but social services representatives did not. There is contact with social services through the Mental Health Forum, but the social services staff who attend this meeting tend not to be senior managers and the Forum is not a decision-making group.

The Trust Board was described as being anxious to listen and as having a good relationship with the group, but they had not been prepared to agree to the request that two service users be appointed to the Board.

All 10 interviewees commented about relationships with people who might be regarded as professional 'allies', but perceptions varied about the extent to which the group was influential within joint forums. The Patients' Council was regarded as a forum in which relationships between service managers and professionals and users were generally positive. One interviewee asserted that the relationship with purchasers was quite friendly, that note was taken of what the group had to say even if they did not act upon it. But one interviewee felt that their role in decision making was minimal, that they had a consultation role but that they were not directly involved in the decision-making process.

A member of the Purchasing for Users Group (PUG) stated: "We work pretty well as a team, it's quite difficult when you first go into these meetings, 'cos they've got the power ... it takes about two or three years to break that down".

He was referring not only to the power to take decisions, but also the power deriving from knowing how the system operates. With increasing emphasis on user involvement PUG wanted the opinions of users more. As an individual he felt that he was treated more as a colleague, but he wondered whether this was because he was a paid employee of the group and was therefore accorded more credibility than someone who could be defined as a 'user'. This is interesting in view of the way in which involvement in a user group can contribute to participants' sense of personal identity (see Barnes and Shardlow, 1996). But it is also an important reflection on the way in which professionals may find it easier to work in partnership with someone who understands the rules of the professional game, rather than seeking to play by the rules of their own game. In other contexts, and if the views being expressed are considered less acceptable, the views of such people may be discounted as 'unrepresentative' and coming from what are referred to as 'professional users'.

The tactics employed by group members in their relationships with officials emphasised persuasion rather than confrontation: "I don't think you really have to shout or threaten"; "I think if we had gone in banging the drum right at the start, we would have been shown the door, the door wouldn't have opened"; "trying to work with people rather than against them".

They described the way in which influence can be achieved through liaising, talking, discussion, communication. This involves persistence and a preparedness to keep returning to an issue in order to achieve a response. This tactic is seen to be strengthened by the pressure on purchasers and providers to be seen to be taking note of users' views, particularly since the group itself is a well-established and well-known user group.

Interviewees believed that the group is in a good position to persuade because they have shown that they are well organised and professional and have a wide variety of people involved rather than one or two outspoken people.

Acceptance of their legitimacy is demonstrated by the fact that professionals refer service users to the advocacy service. One interviewee felt that younger professionals wanted to be more accountable to users and are more sympathetic to the aims and ideals of the group. Another interviewee described the group as having a good relationship with some psychiatrists with the following reservation that illustrates the problems many people with mental health problems experience: "But a lot of people who have mental health problems, they think they're not being believed, and that's sad really. Because they know how they feel". The group has run workshops with psychiatrists and nurses to encourage them to listen to the users of their services more carefully. The group is positively received in such situations. The group had established a very good relationship with the hospital nursing staff who had, on occasion, sought help from the group for projects of their own. One interviewee said: "We're trusted by all sides."

Only two interviewees made comments which suggested that the group might be seen as a threat to managers and professionals. One interviewee described how volunteers could be seen by service providers as just airing grievances and bearing a grudge from the time when they themselves were in hospital.

While the overall picture was of positive relationships, a number of comments suggested a certain frailty. One said of their relationships with purchasers:

"I think it's very thin, very tenuous ... they want a relationship but they don't know what they want from that relationship and I think they are very afraid of that relationship."

Good relationships at a personal level do not disguise the inequality of power. The role of users on joint working groups was often considered to be tokenistic with the power to take decisions or put plans into operation being located within the service purchasers' or providers' groups. Users take part in appointment procedures, but managers retain the right to veto a suggested appointment, although, as we have indicated above, some interviewees recognised that direct involvement in decision making can sometimes be a double-edged sword.

One interviewee noted that the group was not allowed access to management committee minutes of the mental health unit nor to Trust Board minutes. The Trust have not acceded to the group's request for membership of the Board.

"There's been a lot of cosmetic changes but the power balances are still there – around treatment in particular, medication and my position has always been one of challenging that and trying to redress that balance of power."

The impact of the power imbalance was illustrated by reference to the issue of aftercare policy. The group achieved agreement with the purchasers that there should be such a policy and this was devised with a strong input from the group. However, the health authority left it to each provider unit to implement the policy in whatever way was considered appropriate. Consequently in some areas the agreed policy was not fully implemented. The group argued for a consistent aftercare policy for users within PUG but had no success. There was also a dispute over the timing of implementation. Some units were reluctant to put the policy in place immediately, and the suggestion by the group that money should be withheld by the purchasers to the providers until an appropriate policy was in place was not accepted. While one interviewee felt that what had been achieved was a good start, this experience illustrates why some users are reluctant to become participants in a system in which, after considerable effort has been expended, agreements may be compromised because of a lack of power to hold officials to account.

Power imbalances were felt to be exacerbated because of the reliance of the group on statutory agencies for funding, the insecurity of funding, the alien environment in which meetings take place and the language used. Familiarity with such settings increases users' sense of empowerment.

The actual membership of such forums is also very influential and personnel changes can affect the tenor of joint meetings dramatically.

The overall picture that emerged from interviews with activists was of a group that was well established and had earned a considerable degree of respect from many health professionals and managers. Local authority links were less firmly established. The group's links with both users and services enabled it to operate at a strategic level as well as in pursuing specific issues on behalf of individual users. Nevertheless its acceptance as a player within decision-making processes was somewhat precarious. While some power sharing was taking place the power imbalances were still substantial and influence was contingent on successful personal relationships as much as an acceptance of the legitimacy of the group's position within such processes.

Official perceptions of the group's role

Official responses to the group can be considered in regard to three matters:

- the degree to which this group in particular and user groups in general are regarded as legitimate stakeholders in local mental health policy and practice;
- the nature of the role(s) deemed appropriate for such groups; and
- officials' local experience with user groups.

In general terms, and despite some differences of perspective that we report below, there was a great deal of homogeneity in the perceptions expressed by official respondents.

Legitimacy

No respondent offered any principled objection to the recognition of either this particular group or user groups in general as stakeholders who should be heeded and with whom local interactions should be sustained. As one district health authority manager put it:

> **"It is like, it has become the norm to acknowledge the stakeholder. And that one would use them as a source of informal advice that is just as valuable as anybody else's advice. And you are right, we would get shredded if we attempted to do things without them now."**

Since this perception of legitimacy was largely taken to be unproblematic by respondents (subject to some qualifications set out below), it proved difficult to establish what was perceived as its source. One suggestion, from both purchaser and provider managers, was that it reflected practice in the wider world and the growing presence of a national user movement:

"I mean certainly with the development of the user movement nationally, I think there has been a shift. It is now part of accepted customer practice in terms of the philosophy of leading edge organisations."

"And now whereas a decade ago, the idea that you might pay somebody to criticise you was like an alien concept. It is now almost like, again, come into the culture as any healthy organisation that has got nothing to hide except that it needs, that its users need some sort of advocacy, it has to have a complaints procedure, and that you actually get brownie points now for buying advocacy as part of the package."

This implies a managerial role in the growing acceptance of user group activity. Another respondent was more direct: "... when the Chief Executive began to meet with the hospital council and suddenly user involvement became a legitimised activity..."

It also seemed clear that local attitudes to user groups had been influenced by a pivotal event which had occurred a few years before. At a consultative meeting the then management of the health authority had publicly presented plans for the reorganisation of mental health services following the run-down of the local psychiatric hospital. One of our respondents had been present and described what occurred:

"[A woman] who recently joined the CHC, has been very active in the mental health field in [this town], she was in the audience at the back and she just stood up and chaired the meeting and the people on the platform just shrivelled up and died and people turned their chairs round and [she] chaired the rest of the meeting from the back of the room .... the Chief Executive of the Health Authority ... was so appallingly rude to the person who was then Chairman of [the group] – but the [group] contingent stood up and walked out of the meeting ... and with somebody who just on the spur of the moment emerged in the leadership role could organise a meeting and discuss an issue more competently than even these skilled professional officers could..."

One important qualification made by a number of respondents (especially, though not exclusively, psychiatrists) related to the *representativeness* of user groups; they were neither representative of society at large, nor of all users:

> **"I'm not sure that users necessarily represent the society at large. Well in fact I'm sure they don't."**

> **"I think that in collecting the views of users you have to throw your net more widely than just the pressure groups. That you need, that into your audit systems the *user* view and not the *representative's* view, that the actual person there who is using the service at the time." [our emphasis]**

This qualification did not take the form of a denial of user group legitimacy, but reflected genuine tensions for officials in responding to different interests. One tension was that between the civil liberties of people with mental health problems and the public perception of 'dangerous lunatics'. Another was the potential divergence of user and carer interests:

> **"And if you go and talk to some of the groups [other than this group] locally they have a different perspective because they are much more a sort of carers' group than a users' group. And they have quite different perspectives to the users and I think you have to listen to them as well because I think, in providing a service it isn't just for our patients, it is also for the families. And their needs sometimes are different."**

However, potential tensions are not always manifest in practice.

> **"I thought there would be perhaps a lot of potential difficulty around things like admission to hospital, sectioning of people, those kind of issues of civil liberties. And in general I always, the people that I was involved with in general seemed to say there are times when that is the right course of action and it is in the interests of both the individual, the family, the community, whatever that something is done."**

More minor qualifications about the legitimacy of user groups were also raised. One respondent pointed to the potential compromising effect of direct official funding, but recognised that alternative sources were hard to obtain. It was also pointed out that the group manifested a strong white bias (as the group itself recognised):

> **"[The group] has in fact got quite serious limitations in the sense that it doesn't represent all the users. And it particularly doesn't represent the black and Asian group at all. But that is not a problem you see, ... we just meet with their four representatives: that are two paid workers, the chairman and another member of the committee. But through them we've got across to all kinds of other networks."**

However, representativeness was not seen as an overriding problem, but as something which could be managed. A psychiatrist who had raised it as an issue in general went on to dismiss it as a problem so far as the group were concerned: "My experience of them [the group] is that the feedback they give is representative of the sort of things that people say in general".

Nor were local managers seeking one user voice: rather, contacts with organisations such as this seemed to serve as a vehicle for wider networking:

> **"I personally feel that it is a bit dangerous to play games that are about assuming that any one individual representative on the committee or any one organisation that you consult can tell you what user preferences are. It is daft to ask the question because we know it is not a question that can be answered and I personally have found it much more useful to simply use this organisation as a way of networking with a much wider range of people so that you can get a sort of feel for the range of views and preferences and ideas and expectations if they are there, but not to pretend that that can be distilled into one single message."**

Appropriate roles for user groups

Respondents' views about what constituted an appropriate role for this group and for user groups in general focused on roles in relation to the commissioning and provision of health and social care. They did not recognise a role for user groups in a wider context.

'Official' perceptions of appropriate user roles centred around four themes.

First, there was a view that user groups should exist to *challenge professionals*. This view was expressed with varying degrees of acceptance by different respondents. A purchaser (DHA) manager believed that professional autonomy had waned:

> (*Respondent*) **"The days are gone when you get ... a doctor knows better basis. That has kind of gone out of the culture in this building hasn't it?"**

> (*Co-respondent*) **"Oh yes."**

> (*Respondent*) **"Nobody can pull professional rank or anything of that sort any more. You can only, you have to, to some extent, evidence what you are doing or your line of argument and the only credible sort of underpinning line of argument is on the basis of public need, assessed need, community need."**

And yet, the same respondent believed, there was a long way to go before professionals would be prepared to abandon what he described as the 'rituals' of some existing services in favour of much more flexible and informal responses to users' needs.

Several provider respondents expressed the view that even well-meaning and experienced professionals could usefully be challenged from a user perspective. For instance:

> **"But also when I was a social worker and I was having contact with people in [the group] ... on numerous occasions say talking to somebody like — who could just say something and I would think, I'm barking up the wrong tree yet again."**

One manager was concerned that too many challenges could lead to conservative and defensive medicine. But the psychiatrists in our study apparently did not share this reservation or at least did not mention it. One psychiatrist welcomed the existence of user groups as a conduit for complaints that users might feel inhibited in presenting directly to a professional: "Users may tell [group] what they won't tell me because of my white coat for example".

Second, there was a view that user groups ought to *challenge management*. This view was pervasive among respondents, including managers themselves.

> "It is accepted completely by all parties that we can fund them providing they are acting in good faith; they can even slag us off in a public meeting and make the Chief Executive of the Authority look an idiot. Do you know what I mean, that that is not preferred behaviour but that the right is there and that sometimes the necessity might be there?"

> "What strikes me is how – because I remember it – about how arrogant we were 20 years ago into thinking that, the whole power thing, that we knew what people wanted, and they'd have to obey the rules of where they were going to live in our institution and all that. It is incredible now to look back to see how different the world was and how County Hall was in charge. In that sense there is a much more attentive culture that, you know, you ask people what they want."

One professional felt that the recognition of user groups sent a message to *individual* users that dissent was legitimate:

> "My feeling is that the one feeds into the other. That if you've got user groups organised just their existence gives permission to the individuals to put up their hand and say 'I'm not happy with this', you know, because they realise they are in a framework of advocacy."

Another saw a role in helping to avoid further 'scandals' of the kind which had been exposed in long-stay hospitals in the 1960s and 1970s:

> "But if the user group is absent in terms of expressing, you shift back into the pre-1960s... In the seventies I can remember from the Waddington Report institutions which maltreated their patients and institutions which maltreated the citizenry."

Potential challenges to NHS provider management could be made a feature of user involvement in the mechanics of the purchaser/provider split:

"My overall role is quality and quality specifications, monitoring them, and developing them. Within that I conduct monitoring visits to the Trusts and we plan to go to every Directorate there to talk to them about the service and for that we use the user groups and bring them in for a user perspective I suppose, so they can ask their own questions of the service managers and bring their own agenda in."

Third, user groups were felt to have an important *information and education* role. One aspect of this was dispelling myths about mental health, and people with problems, held by both staff and public.

"The popular mythology is that people who really only have got ordinary problems of everyday living yet are labelled as mad or mentally ill and incarcerated in psychiatric hospitals. If you actually go and talk to people their experience is totally different and lots and lots of people at user groups and meetings have talked to me about how the problem isn't that people whisk you into hospital and label you, but that you have to keep banging at the GP's door before anybody will really believe that you've got a serious problem that you need to be in hospital."

The user group had also been regularly employed in a more specific education role: the training of Approved Social Workers (ASWs). The social worker in charge noted that the local authority was

"... bringing the user perspective to sessions in training and we've involved users on both the Approved Social Workers (ASWs) courses I've been involved in and a refresher course I was involved in last October."

Fourth, there was a willingness on the part of both provider managers and professionals to endorse the *participation* of user groups in various decision processes and other activities. For instance, users had been involved in operationalising and monitoring Patients' Charter standards:

"Similarly that centre as well produced a charter for the centre, they've rewritten the quality standards into sort of Patient's Charter stuff to what they would expect as a team. The users were involved in writing them and the user reps

from the user group meet periodically with staff to review
their performance against those expectations."

The group might also be called upon to provide an advocate in patient
case reviews, though this could have dangers in the opinion of one
psychiatrist:

"Well, in our regular [case] reviews we do invite — ... if the
patient wants a user advocate with him, or her, to come. So
I think that can be useful. The danger is that you get so
many people hanging to the roof, you know, the 'does he
take sugar' scenario can be increased rather than mitigated.
You've got so many people that talk about the poor patient
and we try and develop ways of talking which isn't talking
over their heads but it is quite easy actually."

Users were also regularly involved in selecting new members of staff in
NHS establishments. The methods used for this varied in the extent to
which users were integrated into appointments procedures:

"At informal meetings perhaps with lunch or a cup of coffee
or a chat and candidates for the job have to pass through this
informal experience and then somebody ... collates views
and feeds that in. The second approach would be the twin
panel arrangements where staff member would support a
user panel who interview the candidate once and then the
candidate is seen the second time by a staff panel. And the
third approach would be an integrated panel."

Although there had been various problems, including lack of preparation
for user representatives and disagreements over candidates, user
involvement had become routine:

"Statements went out from the then Directorate Manager
saying that we would anticipate users being involved in
interviewing. So it went from being a pioneering initiative
which was available to people who were particularly
enthusiastic about that thing to a general expectation that
everybody should involve the users..."

The same provider manager could see the logic of extending such arrangements to the selection of new entrants to residential places, although this raised dilemmas relating to confidentiality of information about potential residents.

One psychiatrist had also decided to invite the group to participate in a research proposal:

> **"We put in a bid for the [Foundation] and ... I consulted the [group] representative about that and sought his support, and the bid had in it a user evaluation component..."**

In summary, 'official' responses concerning appropriate roles for user groups display the same kind of accepting pragmatism which is evident in their responses about user group legitimacy. User groups have a range of appropriate roles, all of which are being performed locally to some extent. Yet respondents did not make grand claims – as one provider manager said:

> **"That is in its embryonic stage. I think we've got a good track record of involving users at team level in many areas in terms of user forums within the teams involved in care planning and things that relate to the individual particularly but not too good when it comes to the more macro..."**

But in the pluralistic context of health and social care, there are other stakeholders. One psychiatrist summed it up thus:

> **"So the users need to have a voice but certainly not the only voice. And the professionals would like to think that they are able to balance up the voices of the carers, the users, and perhaps society, and maybe some technical things. Whether they do or not I don't know."**

Managerial and professional perceptions of user groups

Local experience of involving users had led to both negative and positive perceptions of this particular group and user groups in general.

Specific criticisms of the group included perceptions that there was internal feuding:

> **"Within [group] there is an enormous amount of feuding**

among the management committee as there is in many small voluntary organisations. There are constant allegations and complaints and grievances about workers who aren't sure who is supposed to be line managing them or who complain that they are never supervised, all those sorts of things, in a way that would not be permitted in any if you like statutory organisation or more formal organisation."

A comment about the resultant stress upon workers was made by a psychiatrist:

"And the small politics that go on between members of the committee once it is set up, can be very difficult to handle because if they've had illness they may have a relapse in illness because of the stresses that they are suffering in the context of their political representation. That has happened a few times."

A psychiatrist felt that the group was often forced into behaving reactively rather than strategically, and sometimes made impractical propositions:

"I think a problem that arises from user involvement is that it is often reactive. It reacts to proposals. It may propose things itself but often because of the lack of expertise it may pose a problem if you like as opposed to a solution. And it is then very hard to take it forward unless you actually bring forward a solution and sometimes when the solutions are put forward they are sometimes impractical."

None of these comments were, however, made in a context of wholly negative opinion; respondents held views which were balanced in several senses. They were balanced with positive comments about this group and in comparison with other user groups, but also balanced with pragmatism; this manager's comments were consonant with the general view which emerged:

"[Group] is actually a chaotic organisation that is very badly managed. If one was to try and describe it as a sort of a theoretical model it is the last thing on earth that one would want anybody else to start imitating or attempting to replicate. But it happens in its eccentric way it works and it meets their needs, and it meets ours. But you couldn't sort of describe it objectively as a model and suggest that some other care group or some other town adopt it... But if the current key personalities there happen to move on to other employment and new people were appointed, I'd anticipate it being completely, absolutely and utterly different and that we would have to alter our style in how we relate to it."

Such comments need to be seen in the context of negative comments about other user groups with whom managers had had dealings. For example:

"And we've got quite a lot of examples of organisations, well again, the — Association is another very good example of an organisation that we fund but isn't functioning terribly well but again has had a weak divided muddled management committee that hasn't managed it properly and we've tried offering sort of advisory input and trying to offer resources to them, trying to indicate that if they want to use any of our services or expertise it is available to them."

The extent of interview material occupied with negative comments about this group is easily outweighed by positive perceptions. The group's 'performance' was highly rated on a number of dimensions, including willingness to be involved, thoroughness of investigation of topics, level of knowledge, ability genuinely to reflect (certain) user opinion, and to communicate effectively, and to work hard:

"I mean in fairness [group] have always been very willing to actually participate given that social worker training, there is no reason why that should be the top of their agenda, there has always been a good response from [group] but having said that, they do have a lot of other commitments and also in user groups inevitably you can't always guarantee that a particular person can be there on a particular day."

"So I think the relationship is good but it can be built on and we can do more I think. And I think [group] itself are stretched ... they have a lot of demands on their time. They've got a number of very committed people down there, but they are all very busy, and they are all doing lots, and so it is about them prioritising their work too and seeing the balance between the individual stuff, which is clearly crucial to the individual but also the macro service which has broad effects on service planning."

"I've been escorted to and shown round projects by users and felt lost, inadequate and supported by the users of [group] because they have a great deal more expertise and knowledge of the place we were visiting. And it was a very salutary experience in that which just continued to remind me that you can't say that this group of people [managers] have got more knowledge, expertise with them just because they've got on a pay roll and others don't because they happen to be using the service."

The generosity of the above judgements, formed by a cross section of professionals and managers, is difficult to interpret as other than the recognition that the group at least is seen as performing a legitimate and useful function. Such an interpretation is supported by several summary comments. First, the group is just another stakeholder, albeit a significant one:

"I think that perhaps the point that I'm trying to make is that our relationship with them is no different to others. It isn't kid gloves, it isn't tokenism, they are just one of the players and they take their chance in the game like everybody else does, and sometimes others are using them and sometimes they are using others and the alliances keep on changing but that is just the way that complex networks and complex organisations operate."

At the same time, an umbrella group such as this had an important role to play in channelling pluralism into a manageable form:

"Yes, it is an umbrella group really which tries to bring together if you like, the representation of these groups I've just described... If they want to feed into say the planning of the services whether this centre would close, or open, or whatever..., they'd find it quite difficult because there isn't directly there isn't any structure for the wider units, the management if you like, to know what the people actually

> feel. So [group] takes over that role and these groups will feed directly into [group] and make their voice heard and then [group] can express it through the city-wide council and various other organisations, community health council. And in that way they build up a political momentum that is sustained for wider political decisions."

Finally, here a provider manager and a psychiatrist voice aspirations for the group's future involvement, visualising a wider and more proactive role:

> "I think that perhaps the challenge for the future is to look at, as I said before, how we can further incorporate [sic] involving them in looking at how we sort of plan at a more macro level."

> "We've been providing them with minutes and more recently we've been providing them with a sort of summary of the minutes and we're going to start supplying them with agendas before the meetings so that they can, if they want to, raise items on the agenda."

Motivations to enhance the involvement of the group within decision-making processes include an instrumental aspect which we have described elsewhere as 'strategic userism' or 'playing the user card' (Harrison et al, 1997):

> "The card you have to play all the time is user need, user preference and user view on something and whether I am negotiating with other people inside this building, arguing with the provider Trust, negotiating with the social services department, arguing about how we ought to spend joint finance, no matter what I'm doing you do in effect play the user card."

Conclusion

This group has adopted a strategy based largely on working with officials and their legitimacy in this respect has broadly been accepted by those officials. Nevertheless a number of comments from officials suggest that such legitimacy is contingent on a perceived acceptability of the position taken by the group, and could be undermined if different (more radical?) positions were taken. Official perceptions of internal organisational weaknesses are interesting in this respect. The user group appears to be judged on its capacity to conform to practice in formal organisations (viz the reference to line management) when such criteria may be neither appropriate nor relevant to a group with a very different nature and purpose.

Relationships have built up over many years and many of the key players within the group had been constant during that time. For the group this raises questions about its capacity to respond to and reflect the aspirations of younger people with mental health problems. For example, another of the mental health user groups in our study focused its energies particularly on responding to younger people's needs and had taken a decision *not* to engage in changing mainstream services, but to set up an alternative resource. On the other hand, this experience meant that group members between them had developed a considerable resource of knowledge and skills which were clearly significant in winning respect and credibility from officials. Key players in the user group had longer experience of mental health services in the city than many of the officials with whom they were working.

Separate organisation by users has been a vital means of sustaining relationships with officials during this period, as well as enabling a widening of the net in terms of those involved. Some described how they had been encouraged to take on roles within centre or sector groups and subsequently had been supported in taking on broader roles within the group.

The tensions revealed in this study are thus similar to those experienced by other social movements which gain maturity and some official acceptance for their views. They are then in danger of losing the radical edge which provided the initial motivation and which may be necessary to engage younger people whose experiences have been forged within different contexts from those of the movement's founders.

FOUR

Implementing the social model of disability – after the honeymoon

Movements with objectives for social change may have to face up to the dilemmas of success as well as the need to adapt to changing circumstances. If a movement is built on opposition what happens when the ideas it seeks to promote start to become accepted into mainstream thinking? Feminists working in the Women's Refuge Movement, for example, had to make decisions about their preparedness to work within State institutions once the reality of male violence had been accepted as a legitimate focus for action by local authorities (Lovenduski and Randall, 1993). But they also had to address the fact that ideas themselves can undergo change in the process.

The disability movement can claim considerable success in shifting thinking about the nature of disablement. Disability rights legislation is now on the statute book and the media are scrutinising images of disabled people for their tendencies to portray 'tragic heroes' or 'objects of pity'. Disabled people are more visible within public spaces because those public spaces are more accessible to them. While disability activists would rightly claim that they are far from fully achieving the objectives of the movement, many would also acknowledge that they face new dilemmas as a result of the opportunities to enter into more formal relationships with powerful decision makers (eg Barnes and Oliver, 1995).

The disabled people's organisation which is the subject of this chapter is the longest established coalition in the country. Members include activists who have contributed substantially to the thinking of the movement nationally and internationally, and it is based within a local authority area which prides itself on its radical equal opportunities policies. Yet interviews revealed that some members of the Coalition were not optimistic about its future role vis-à-vis local health and social services agencies. In this chapter, as well as describing the nature and objectives of the group from the perspectives of those active within it, we will consider the nature of changes which have taken place within the Coalition's relationship with statutory agencies from the perspectives of both 'sides'. Such changes need to be understood by reference to particular characteristics of the local situation, but also to the substantial changes which have taken place in the ideology and structure of welfare discussed in Chapter 1.

Origins of the Coalition

The Coalition was established in 1981, the International Year of Disabled People (IYDP). Organisations of disabled people were already active alongside more traditional voluntary organisations in the area. A disability information service (DIAL) was run by disabled volunteers with a grant from the county council, and UPIAS – the Union of Physically Impaired Against Segregation – was also active. The event which sparked off the formation of the Coalition was the exclusion by able-bodied organisers of these disabled people's groups from involvement in planning local events to mark the IYDP. Together with the social services department, DIAL organised a separate conference to mark IYDP, with its central theme 'full participation and equality'. In order to pursue this theme the conference decided to form a coalition along similar lines to organisations already operating in North America – a democratically organised body under the control of disabled people, with a belief that disabled people themselves must be the prime movers in the fight for self-determination and equality.

Constitution, structure and funding

The Coalition is a representative democracy. Members are invited to make nominations for election to the 15-member council. Voting on these nominations is by postal ballot, with the vote ratified and endorsed at the Annual General Meeting. Officers of the council are elected by council members. Only disabled people are allowed to vote and hold office, although able-bodied people can become associate members and attend the AGM. Representatives to participate in consultation or planning meetings with service providers are chosen at monthly council meetings. These representatives are expected to report back to the council on a regular basis.

At the time of interviews (September 1994) the Coalition employed a part-time administrative assistant, a part-time clerical support worker, and a publicity and information officer on a short-term contract. Many people work for the organisation on a voluntary basis. Before substantial reductions in funding (see below) the Coalition had been able to employ more people.

The Coalition is committed to the integration of able-bodied and disabled people and seeks to reflect this in its employment policy. Thus, it has an equal opportunities statement, although a policy of affirmative action is used to select between able-bodied and disabled candidates with equal qualifications.

The county council has always been the main funder of the Coalition. In 1981 it provided £20,000 grant aid. This increased prior to charge capping (restrictions placed by the then Conservative government on the amount local authorities could raise through the community charge) to £50,000. In 1994 the Coalition received £24,000 from the county council and a smaller amount from a district council. It received no money from the health authorities, although between 1983 and 1985, when the (then) Centre for Independent Living was being planned (see below), a community link worker post was funded through joint finance.

Uncertainty over funding means lack of security for employees and a constant need to seek out and apply for new funding. Reliance on volunteers and those with demonstrated capabilities to take on the work of the Coalition can lead to enormous pressures on individuals. Decisions about which issues are adopted as priorities for action can be determined less by "the organisation's philosophical or political analysis of what ought to be prioritised" as by what they are required to deal with in order to retain their credibility, and even their existence.

Membership

Full membership is open to anyone identifying themselves as a disabled person. Membership implies acceptance of the basic aims of the Coalition and people can be expelled if they are no longer able to accept these. Membership is open to organisations as well as to individuals, and members of those organisations who are disabled can vote in elections. There is a strong emphasis on the openness and democratic nature of the Coalition, and on ensuring broad membership from all disability groups.

Membership numbers have fluctuated during the life of the Coalition between approximately 300 and 900. The majority of interviewees wanted the Coalition to be as broad-based an organisation as possible, although there was a recognition of the reluctance of some disabled people to become members of what was seen to be a political organisation. One spoke of the wish to ensure that the Coalition was capable of embodying

"... this collective experience of exclusion and we want to be

> able to represent it at every level from the very simple local
> level ... to the developed political awareness of activists and
> all stages in between."

The significance of size in relation to credibility was also recognised:

> "When I go down to Whitehall or to the county offices or
> the health authority and knock on their door, I represent X
> number of members, so I think it is important. I think it's
> good to have people at the back of you, because through
> unity you've got strength."

But activists acknowledged the tension between being a broadly based
coalition and maintaining a clear identity based in a commitment to
key principles.

> "You meet the resistance of people who don't want to get
> political. That's one of the barriers and there are these key
> points where the way you express yourself, usually when you
> start to get really enthusiastic and suggest how powerful this
> sort of sharing and coming together can be, you actually put
> off the very people whose experience you value and want to
> bring into the organisation. I don't know what the key to
> that is. I've never found it!"

> "You've got on one hand the weight of received ideas about
> disability that influence all people's minds whether able or
> disabled, but when it's disabled people battling, having to
> accept or receive ideas that are very different and
> uncomfortable, challenging and dangerous, that it's no wonder
> that people are not flocking to join."

The Coalition seeks to make connections between personal experiences
of disability and a political analysis of these experiences, but acknowledges
that such understanding cannot be forced and that some people will
always be reluctant to join an overtly political organisation:

> "From time to time you do get very specifically focused
> groups who are impatient with other disabled people for
> their failure to see the nature of their oppression but this
> really is something that people have to take at their own

pace. If you don't, if you just adopt the words, then it's all false and it all starts to revolve around nonsense about political correctness and general attitudinising rather than real understanding of oppression."

Criticisms that the Coalition was too male–dominated led to the establishment of a women's group. However, in common with the mental health group discussed in the previous chapter, the Coalition has found it difficult to involve black disabled people, although one of our interviewees was Asian. One reason for lack of success in engaging with minority ethnic groups was felt to be the distance from the Coalition's office base and the city in which the majority of people from minority ethnic groups lived. Lack of resources also meant limited opportunities to translate material into minority languages.

The Coalition was also experiencing difficulty recruiting younger members. One member wondered whether the lack of involvement of younger people was a sign of success of integration policies: "maybe they are doing their own thing in the community and why should they label themselves as disabled".

A younger disabled people's group had been started and, at the time of writing, a youth development post was being recruited to address the involvement of younger people.

There was concern that disabled people whose identities also derived from their sexuality or membership of a minority ethnic group may find their concerns marginalised within the Coalition:

"It is not that it has been excluding these groups because it is built into the constitution that all people are welcomed ... but again you have to have something on offer to these groups ... it is about opening the membership up and saying what are the things you want to read about and what are the things you want to hear about. How can we campaign on your behalf, how can we get involved?"

One interviewee also suggested that class was a factor in limiting membership. He thought that a progressive and radical group like the Coalition would not be attractive to middle class and upper class individuals.

The absence of people with hearing impairments from the Coalition was noted. The general feeling was that members of this group were already organising themselves around their own identity, experience and culture and consequently had little time to become involved in the wider movement. One interviewee also observed that a hearing impaired council member was having considerable difficulty lip-reading and he then realised that all the male members of the council had beards and moustaches which effectively hid their lips.

Attempts were being made to involve people with learning disabilities. A person with a learning disability had become a member of the council and attempts were being made to ensure that documents produced by the Coalition were suitably written. One interviewee also mentioned the possibility that people with mental health problems might become members.

However, whether or not individual disabled people become members of the Coalition, interviewees were agreed that it exists not just to serve the interests of its members, but of all disabled people.

Objectives, activities and influence

The Coalition was founded on two fundamental principles:
- that it should be a democratic, grass-roots organisation, controlled by securing the active participation of disabled people; and
- that disability should be understood as a social phenomenon.

> **We believe the most effective policies are ones which attack the root causes of disability. Our view is that these root causes are to be found in society. For this reason Coalition policy is directed out into society, and aims to promote awareness and take actions which remove social and physical barriers and thus overcome disability. (Coalition policy document)**

It aims to embrace all impairments by emphasising the common experience of disability within the public domain, rather than the personal and different experiences of people which arise from different types of impairments. It aims to move away from the traditional view of individual disabled people's needs, to a consideration of the way that society needs to change in order to secure full participation and equality for all. Problems are to be defined by disabled people themselves rather than by able-bodied professionals. Disabled people's participation in the decision-making process of central and local government should be developed.

All of the Coalition's practical projects are located within the theoretical framework defined by the social model of disability. This framework has been applied to the analysis of a broad range of issues including: the relationship between lack of equal opportunities and low self-esteem among disabled people; whether the presumed physical condition of a foetus should be accepted as sufficient reason for abortion; the relationship between disability and war; the design of the built environment; and responses to the Patient's Charter.

The social model of disability represents an entirely different perspective on the notions of 'care' and 'welfare' from those contained within most formal policy statements regarding community care. It thus constitutes a challenge to professional career structures within welfare agencies. Disabled people are represented not as dependants in need of care, but as citizens with rights to participate alongside and with able-bodied people. The first aim of the Coalition is "to promote the active participation of disabled people in securing the greatest possible independence in daily living activities, full integration into society, and full control over their lives." (Aims and Policy document). While providers of health services have a role to play in providing the general and particular health services which disabled people need, and social services have a role in providing aids and adaptations, personal care assistants, and some information and advice services, the social model implies that neither health nor social services authorities should have a role in providing residential or day care for disabled people. Hence much of the Coalition's energies have been directed towards *limiting* the role of social care agencies as service providers and campaigning for resources to be invested in supporting the integration of disabled people into mainstream social life. From this perspective, the roles of architects, engineers, planners and designers may be more significant than those of social workers, residential or day care managers, or community nurses.

The Coalition's aims include: improving employment opportunities; improving disabled people's access to the built environment; achieving legislative change concerned with anti-discrimination and rights to services; and influencing the public's perception of disabled people, particularly by means of media portrayals. They are also concerned with improving access to educational and training opportunities and to leisure services, and increasing disabled people's participation in politics. Many of these objectives are pursued in alliance with others involved in the disability movement and in some instances with other social movements.

From the start the Coalition has been involved in practical projects designed to support integration in different ways. For example, signing classes were held to improve communication between hearing and hearing impaired people, disabled people were helped to set up in business, and an access survey was carried out. The aims included in the Coalition's policy document also refer to campaigning to achieve accessible transport, support for continued moves towards the integration of disabled people into the education system, and support for measures to achieve equal work opportunities "whether by integration into the workplace of ordinary employment or by developing full equivalent home-working alternatives".

A good example of the way in which disabled people's expertise can assist professionals to fulfil their obligations was the agreement, early in the Coalition's life (1983/84), that all planning applications for public buildings would come to the Coalition who would have them scrutinised for their accessibility by disabled architects.

Similarly, the Coalition's objective in relation to housing is that all new build housing should conform to specifications which would enable access to disabled people. The 'Access for Life' campaign has focused on ensuring that all new housing is built to the Coalition's 'accessible–adaptable' standards. The aim is to introduce

"... design specifications which mean that you start off with a housing unit which is a good general access on the assumption that in its lifetime – 100 years or whatever – it's bound to be used by a certain proportion of disabled occupants and a larger number of disabled visitors."

Activists described a 'productive tension' between the pursuit of practical projects and the development of ideas, and also a tension between acting on priorities identified by the Coalition, and reacting to events taking place both locally and nationally. They utilise a variety of strategies to pursue their objectives.

Joint working

The representation of disabled people within key decision-making forums is both an end in itself and a means to achieving other objectives. All interviewees believed that the Coalition should aim to participate in service planning. All but one believed that it should be involved in monitoring and evaluation, and in decision making about priorities and resource allocation. Seven of the nine interviewees thought it should participate in service management.

The biggest single practical project with which the Coalition has worked with the county council, has been the establishment of what was originally known as a Centre for Independent Living and subsequently called a Centre for *Integrated* Living (CIL). The difference is important. The concept of 'independent living' emphasises the aim of individual choice equivalent to choices available to the general population, and also the rights of individuals to have their needs met. *Integrated* living emphasises the full participation of disabled people within the community. It is seen as having a collective rather than individualistic emphasis through the objective of enabling community participation, as well as enabling disabled people to live independent lives in the way they choose. It emphasises the responsibilities as well as the rights of citizenship, and mutuality as well as independence. However, the term 'integration' has caused some difficulties for black disabled people who seek to emphasise self-determination rather than integration.

In 1982 a joint working party was established to work with the county council towards the establishment of the CIL. The CIL model provided a focus for the redirection of existing services towards achieving integrated living. In spite of opposition from some professionals the county council agreed to fund the CIL. The constitution of the CIL was agreed in 1984 and in 1985 it was set up as an autonomous independent company. Half of the members of the general council of the CIL are appointed by the Coalition and half by the county council. The involvement of disabled and able-bodied people on the general council and the employment of disabled and able-bodied people within the centre are both seen as examples of the integration which is the centre's overall objective.

Agreement to establish the CIL was accompanied by negotiations which led to the closure of a day centre and a hostel for disabled people. In addition to producing a different model of services, this experience provided a practical demonstration of disabled people as decision makers capable of creating alternative service models and taking greater control over their lives.

Interviewees considered that the constitutional relationship between the Coalition and the CIL is clear. However, there has sometimes been a lack of clarity at operational level and not all officials have understood the relationship:

> **"They see the same people involved and they can't understand that we wear different hats ... they can't understand that one is a campaigning membership organisation and the other is**

> **a non-membership organisation which provides services, but managed by the same people. That's been very difficult, it has been a difficult animal to manage."**

After the establishment of the CIL the Coalition had to re-establish its priorities:

> **"A lot of people felt at the time that once we'd done that the Coalition would go out of existence because they felt that was all that we had been set up to do. It wasn't, but all our energy went into it for about two years and after that we had to look at ourselves and say, well, now what do we do and we realised that there was a lot of things that had been neglected. And even when we got CIL we were then managers and we'd got to learn all those skills as well."**

The 1990 NHS and Community Care Act necessitated further review of the way in which the Coalition should work with statutory agencies. One of the Coalition objectives is that

> **"... the means should exist for democratically organised groups of representatives of disabled people to be involved in the way services are developed and the way they are run. (Consultation policy document)**

Opportunities for disabled people's input into community care planning processes were seen as a means of pursuing this objective. This has included input on disabled people's consultative groups, on planning groups within the social services committee structure, on advisory groups, as well as regular informal meetings with social service managers. Because the county is large and services are organised on a locality basis the nature of involvement may be different in different areas.

One person spoke of the personal dilemmas and experience associated with her involvement as chair of a local planning group:

> **"It's difficult knowing which hat to wear, me as an individual, but hopefully I represent the four – me as an individual first and foremost, as a worker of CIL and the Coalition and also as an activist. My experience is coming from all that and trying to actually implement all that and you are not sure as a worker just how far you should push the situation, how far**

should you go and that can be a bugbear, but then at the end of the day as a disabled person, as an individual in my own right, then sod it ... then you know you get the feeling of isolation, you know, is it just me, why aren't there more people like me saying the same thing?"

Involvement in planning had been an objective from the early days of the Coalition and early successes had come about as a result of effective work within joint planning groups before the requirement to consult over community care plans. However, the proliferation of bodies with some planning remit in both purchaser and provider agencies, and the development of locality planning led to increasing demands on those who have developed expertise in working with those bodies. One person felt: "These opportunities to get on to advisory groups, consultative groups and planning groups develop faster than the expertise and ability to respond to them".

Influence has also been sought through involvement with Community Health Councils, and through involvement as lay inspectors in inspection procedures introduced by the 1990 Act.

Joint working within the health and social care system is intended to lead to service change of direct benefit to all disabled people. One example of this was the development of an independent living flat for people who had never previously lived independently. Examples of issues pursued with health services were more to do with access to facilities than with the nature of the services themselves. They included: the lack of parking bays for disabled people attending hospital clinics; poorly printed appointment letters that visually impaired people had difficulty in reading; and reception desks that were too high for people in wheelchairs. The women's group raised the issue of access to mammography units which they say had 'planned out' disabled women.

Enabling individual disabled people to take on the management of their own carers has been an important objective. One interviewee recalled the impact on local authority representatives of an American disabled woman who came to talk about control over personal assistants by disabled people. "I guess for the first time they began to understand that someone in a wheelchair can have some control".

But securing individual control over personal support services was considered to offer advantages to the local authority as well as to disabled people themselves:

"We actually believe that the participatory model of service

provision brings economies, prevents waste, prevents very
elaborate segregative, long-term provisions being set up where
supports and encouragements to quite short-term
developments to get people back into managing their own
lives could happen instead."

Research, training and alternative models

The Coalition's strategy is founded on a commitment to the social
model of disability. In practice that can involve "getting society to
think differently and give better provision rather than raise money to
find cures", or "trying to introduce into the minds of the people who
are being trained the ideas that are coming from the disabled people's
movement".

It does not involve setting up an alternative service structure outside
the state welfare system:

"In the UK where you have already got a very elaborate
welfare system, you're not going to set up an alternative,
we're not going to be able to set up as a ragged school of
service provision in a way that alternative education was set
up 100 years ago. So progress does depend on existing public
service providers slowly changing their idea of their role."

Commitment to the social model is reflected in the Coalition's
contribution to research through which the implications of the model
can be explored and developed, and training through which it can impact
on professional practice. Members are continually monitoring and
evaluating services through contact with disabled people who use them.
The Coalition has also been involved in more formal research projects
undertaken directly or through collaboration with research institutes
and universities. Several interviewees remarked that the Coalition had
never had the resources to conduct 'significant research', although they
were considering applying for a research grant. A pilot study was being
conducted by a university researcher into the needs of younger disabled
people in one area of the county and it was hoped that this might lead
to funding for a more significant project.

Training is a significant part of the Coalition's activities and is often
undertaken in collaboration with the CIL. Much of this is focused on
front-line workers such as social workers and home helps. Coalition

members are very aware that disability awareness training often flies in the face of professional training:

> **"It's a very big job because it actually reverses the thrust of several years' training in many cases. It's not easy working with a colleague newly arrived in social services full of enthusiasm and idealism to say that the training that produced those ideas – just forget it!"**

But there was also evidence that officials welcomed the informal learning which came from working with disabled people:

> **"Elected officers who have worked alongside us for some time now are saying, 'We've learned a lot from you, it has been a privilege to work with you and we now understand a lot more about disability than we ever did before.'"**

One person expressed caution about the need to ensure that front-line workers who were themselves comparatively powerless within service systems should not be exploited as a result of the introduction of new service models which involve a shift in power between providers and recipients:

> **"I was concerned about the home helps, I was concerned that if the bounds were chipped too far that these women, who had very little power, could be exploited. Although as I said, there were lots of assurances of course that this wouldn't happen and that people wouldn't be treated like that. And I think that the difficulty was weighing up the needs of the individual, of both groups, carers – the providers – and the people who required to live independently."**

The Coalition's national standing in contributing to both theory and practice is well recognised. They have been involved in the publication of many papers and have produced part of a unit for the Open University Social Problems and Social Welfare Course.

Using the market

The Coalition aims to achieve change in the nature of services provided within the welfare state, not to propose an alternative structure. The

CIL has been the main practical expression of a model in which disabled people are active partners in service provision.

As we have indicated, there was reluctance to give credence to the health and social care market by supporting the mechanisms to which it had given rise. All but one of our interviewees felt that the Coalition should aim to participate in service purchasing, but no one chose this as a priority. Nevertheless, eight interviewees believed that the Coalition should aim to enable individual disabled people to purchase their own services directly and four people saw this as a priority:

> **"One of the things we have always tried to develop is to enable people to have control over money, to get money in their hand and to buy the kind of service that they feel is appropriate."**

The general feeling was that this would take place through the CIL which is actively involved in assisting disabled people to employ their own personal assistants. In addition a contract had been agreed with the local authority for the CIL to employ care assistants to provide support to people in their own homes.

In discussing the way in which the relationship between the Coalition and the CIL could be seen to mirror the provider/purchaser split one person recognised that this implied

> **"... signing up to this notion of introducing markets into public services which nobody consulted disabled people about and it would never have occurred to the organisation of disabled people that we revert to ideas that were dumped in our grandparents' time."**

The most significant issue to emerge from interview responses was that of control rather than ownership of services. While there was little evidence that Coalition members welcomed the introduction of the market into health and social services, the opportunities provided by the market to enable disabled people to exercise more control over personal support services were being used.

Campaigning and politics

As a leading member of the disability movement in the UK and internationally, the Coalition has a strong political identity. It is prepared to work both within and outside the official system to pursue its objectives.

A proactive campaigning style was evident in the campaign for the CIL and also campaigns about social security benefits and for disabled people to have control over their own personal assistants. Coalition members played a large part in national campaigns for anti-discrimination legislation, organising deputations to Westminster as well as local events to raise awareness and seek support for the Bill, and letter writing to MPs.

The Coalition has also had to adopt a reactive stance in relation to, for example, certain local access issues, and skin-toned hearing aids for black disabled people.

Campaigning methods include using the media, producing their own newsletter and other publications, negotiation and "barging into meetings".

Direct action is not the preferred option: "At the end of the day ... it's far better to jaw, jaw, jaw than go to war, war, war. But if it has to we shall". One example of this was when a group of about 12 people had 'stormed' a conference organised by the health authority to discuss sex and sexuality of disabled people to which no disabled people had been invited.

The Coalition has supported people who have been involved in direct action and they are affiliated to the Direct Action Network. They have campaigned against events such as Telethon which portray disabled people as recipients of charity.

Members have campaigned to stop the development of land which would have hindered disabled people's access to the countryside. This would have led to direct action – a mass trespass – if their initial campaign had not been successful:

> **"The first day you shut that off and you put a security guard there, that'll be the day that we shall go through. That is the day you will be arresting us. That is the day you will be carting us off to prison."**

One interviewee saw direct action as an important way of raising awareness and of presenting a positive image of disabled people:

> **"I have listened to all the arguments for and the reasons why and the reasons why not and now my personal thing is it is**

time to change and again to bring about that change then,
for me, direct action is the only way forward for that."

This man was involved with the Direct Action Network and had
demonstrated against faith healers, charity appeals, transport issues and
at anti-discrimination legislation rallies. He had been arrested. But he
had also seen immediate changes taking place – a cinema had introduced
access for disabled people within a few days of a demonstration. He
had found direct action important personally:

"It takes away some of the anger and frustration that you are
feeling and you change that around then to empowerment
of disabled people. You get a thrill and a buzz from that."

However, another interviewee felt equally strongly that direct action
was not for her. She believed that many other disabled people had been
alienated from the movement because of the use of direct action. She
was not sure

"...that people take any notice ... for me it feels like people
out there are saying 'Oh, it's them again'. And I'm not sure
we are getting the right message over with public
demonstration."

She made the point that for many disabled people

"...it is not a safe arena to be in either. I've got brittle bones,
I'd be terrified at being arrested and being thrown into a
van."

She felt her views on this had been respected within the organisation.
These two very different perspectives demonstrate the range of views
within the Coalition about the tactics which should be adopted to
achieve their objectives. It embraces very different views and provides
opportunities for people to act in different ways in the pursuit of common
objectives.

Relationships with service providers

The Coalition was formed long before the rhetoric of consumerism
become influential within health and social care services. During the

mid-1980s the group had been able to establish itself as an influential body in relation to a county council which was keen to demonstrate radical credentials. But the advent of 'user involvement' as a more widely accepted policy objective was not considered to have enhanced the position of the Coalition. One interviewee reflected on this:

> **"By having disabled people active and around for a while, it's no longer new, it's no longer to be looked on as an interesting phenomenon, it's no longer to be looked on ... as reflecting well on the county council for its perspicacity in assisting, financial assistance for the organisation to come into being. That honeymoon period has gone. What it has been replaced with is something much more sticky and difficult."**

This change in the nature of the relationship between the Coalition and the county council was attributed in part to changes in the relationship between central and local government which placed financial and other constraints on the county council; and in part to the implementation of community care legislation which had been driven by the thinking of a new right Tory government.

The emphasis on individualism rather than collectivism within welfare was considered to have redefined Coalition objectives away from collective action to achieve social change:

> **"The hardest thing to have to come to terms with, I think, is the reassessment of the role of the individual as distinct from the role of society; the balance between these two seems to have changed in a way that isn't easy to make sense of in terms of future outcomes."**

This interviewee felt that the campaign for anti-discrimination legislation was a feature of this move to an emphasis on individual rights rather than the "historical process of collective action to achieve change." (We discuss the significance of this in the context of different views of 'community care' in Barnes et al, 1998.)

Coalition members who had been involved from the start provided a historical perspective on the way in which relationships had developed.

Prior to the establishment of the Coalition, UPIAS had challenged council policy on segregated accommodation, while DIAL had had contact with the social services department's development section and had made an input to local authority conferences at which alternative service developments were being discussed.

In 1982 the Coalition encouraged the county council to endorse a Statement of Intent on disability policy signed by all main committees. This stated the council's intention to aim for full participation and equality of opportunity; to involve disabled people actively on all advisory and consultative committees; to create a barrier-free built environment; and to develop integrated independent living arrangements, an accessible public transport system, integrated education, and dissemination of information. Membership was obtained on sub-committees and monitoring groups of social services and CHCs. The Coalition was involved in the development of the local authority equal opportunities policy.

Changes in the planning structures introduced as a result of the NHS and Community Care Act caused the Coalition to reconsider its role. For example, in the past both the Coalition and the CIL were represented in joint planning teams. Should the Coalition now seek to develop relationships with commissioners (purchasers) while the CIL worked more closely with providers? There was a reluctance to be 'shoved into' roles to fit the planning structures being developed by statutory agencies, and the introduction of the purchaser/provider split was seen as being unhelpful to the Coalition:

"This distinction between planning and purchasing bodies and providing bodies is an added obstacle to us because it means we have to prioritise and spread ourselves more thinly and select where representation is going to be most effective."

Decisions about where to place priorities and invest energies thus become more important and more difficult.

The Coalition also had representation on bodies such as the Rural Development Council, Police Consultative Committees, and Community Education Councils. Such commitments were reviewed in the light of other demands on members' time and a decision made to maintain this representative role, although a dissenting view was expressed that the Coalition should be emphasising its campaigning role rather than seeking to maintain involvement in these various forums.

The development of the CIL increased contacts with disabled people who were not members of the Coalition. This led the Coalition to consider the extent to which it should engage with groups which are not members. The county council questioned the Coalition's ability to speak as the representative voice of disabled people in the county since there were some groups which were not members of the Coalition. Two very different views on the issue of 'representative' are evident here. The Coalition bases its claim to representativeness on the fact that council members are elected by other disabled people – a model which reflects the legitimacy with which members of the county council can claim to speak as representatives of their constituents. The county council argued that a 'representative' body would consist of members from all the different groups claiming to represent disabled people, since this would reflect the differences of view evident among those groups. This corporatist model would also, presumably, leave the county council in the position of being able to choose for itself which of those differing views it would respond to. A county-wide Disabled People's Forum was established at local authority instigation in order to provide what it considered to be a more representative group of disabled people with whom the council could consult. The Coalition considered the Forum to be undemocratic and not a grass-roots organisation. Initially it operated a policy of non-cooperation but later became involved from time to time depending on its perceived priority in comparison with other activities.

A number of interviewees talked about changes in the level of funding received from the county council and reflected on what this meant for the Coalition and for its relationship with the local authority. Some of those involved at the time the cuts were made regarded these as a political action designed to 'clip the wings' of the Coalition, although not all saw this as discriminatory action since voluntary bodies generally experienced cuts in their grants when rate-capping was introduced.

One interviewee suspected that fear of losing local authority funding caused the Coalition to tone down its approach. He suggested there had been a split of opinion within the group as to whether they should become more political or whether they should "go back to being a little more cap in hand".

As well as the direct impact of reductions in grant aid, financial restrictions on the local authority were considered to have had a detrimental effect on the nature of services provided by the authority: "The services have become so narrow that they are being designed by able-bodied people and they are just being inflicted on us again".

This in turn made it more difficult for the Coalition to develop confidence among disabled people to challenge service providers to be more accountable.

The nature of the relationship between the Coalition and service providers and purchasers was seen by one interviewee as "tokenistic – for political reasons they have to be seen to be doing something". However, another felt that the important thing was to be involved and to acknowledge that there were bound to be complications within relationships with 'officials'. Another felt that it was important to establish a partnership with the authorities:

> **"I wouldn't want people to run away with the idea that we would block everything. That's why I would say yes, if the professionals would come and meet us, we would meet them and I would find that a way of partnership down the middle."**

Individual factors have affected relationships with both social services and health services:

> **"We would want to work alongside social services ... but I never had much to do with him [the Director] because I just didn't seem to speak his language. But — [the Deputy Director] I could and we used to meet quite frequently and we'd talk about these issues that would crop up."**

One interviewee spoke of a hospital consultant:

> **"He's a good contact to have ... we can learn from his professional skills and, you know, he can take on board some of our attitudes when dealing with a patient."**

Interviewees reflected on other ways in which the nature of relationships had changed. At first:

> **"The county council never stopped us ... they were very helpful towards us. You know, let's know what the teething problems are, and what the problems are, we'll try and iron them out."**

> **"We have had a lot of support in the past from non-disabled professionals, you know, like OTs and social workers, people like that. We particularly had a lot of support in our growth period, right at the beginning."**

Some interviewees were sceptical about this, and thought that the council wanted to be seen to be doing "the right thing" . Another felt that the novelty value of the Coalition had been lost because it had been around for some time:

> **"That honeymoon period has gone. What it has been replaced with is something much more difficult because ... firstly because I think of uncertainties within the authority, political and with senior officers about the role of the authority and its political orientation and partly because of the preoccupations of the authority and its officers and members with the technicalities of having to introduce legislation that has been forced upon them."**

However, another interviewee felt that the Coalition had presented a threat to professionals in its early days:"When the Coalition came along, professionals said, 'What's going on! We've never had to put up with this before! We had full control.'"

As we have noted, the social model of disability does represent a threat to those professionals who are unwilling or unable to develop their practice in response to the different insights offered by this analysis. The issue of control includes the fundamental question of who defines what is legitimate knowledge.

Another view was that the relationship between the Coalition and officials was one of growing respect:

> **"I think we've gained a lot of respect from people over the years... Elected officers who have worked alongside us for some time now are saying, 'We've learned a lot from you, it has been a privilege to work with you and we now understand a lot more about disability than we ever did before'."**

> **"In the early days it was all anger, banner waving, occasionally disrupting meetings, now thanks to long-standing members like — and — and others, relationships have been struck up between [the Coalition] and the county council and health authorities."**

Another interviewee echoed this:

> **"They're actually beginning to see that direct experience is worth taking note of, because it benefits them as far as running**

the services efficiently and cheaply and giving us a better standard of service."

The Coalition has changed too:

"We can learn from each other. I think we have learnt from them as well, we have learnt how to negotiate, we've learnt a lot of skills from them, we've learnt a few crafty tricks from them as well! Like walking out of meetings in the middle and things like that!"

There was a view that the Coalition's successes in its early period had been a factor in the reduction of its funding from the local authority:

"I think the day of the long knives had been out for some while... And that's why the Coalition had its wings clipped because we would tread on people's toes, not deliberately, but to make sure ... you see, able-bodied people like to think they know everything about disabled people. It was good for their ego ... when you were going to get elected it's nice to put on your little bit of manifesto that I did this for disabled people. So I think some able-bodied people found themselves threatened now because of the power of the Coalition."

There was also a sense of growing fear from local authorities:

"I think they are afraid, I really think they are afraid of the mass move among disabled people ... I think they are worried about the anti-discrimination legislation because they know that once we have got it we will go all out to make it work and they know that it is going to cost them."

One suggested this sense of threat was intensified by the Coalition's standing within the national disability movement.

These descriptions of the shifts in the relationship between the Coalition and local officials reflect the significance of power within that relationship as well as changes in the political and resource context. The descriptions of interactions with the local authority indicate an attitude of 'so far and no more' on the part of officials to the Coalition's attempts to influence services and decision-making processes. Disabled people are not represented as of right within consultative and decision-making forums. Representation has to be offered by the authorities or won by the Coalition. Years of work and negotiation could be lost if one person changes their job, or because the local authority is obliged to bring in new systems.

The official view

There is no doubt that at the time of the research the Coalition and the CIL were seen by officials as credible political actors and the focus of a collective, campaigning voice for disabled people's rights as citizens. This perception was shared by all but one of the officials interviewed and held particularly strongly by local government people. This reflects the special, historical relationship between the Coalition and later the CIL and the county council and district council which had provided funding for the Coalition. Politicians and some officers saw the ascendance of the Coalition in the context of the 'halcyon days' of Left Labour council power in the late 1970s and early 1980s, before the arrival of compulsory competitive tendering and the 1990 NHS and Community Care Act. There was a sense that this is now a lost domain of liberality in which community education, the local peace movement and large-scale support for the disabled people's Coalition once flourished simultaneously. Years later these movements seem to have become conflated, partly because all have now been marginalised. In the context of a strong tradition of political activism in the county, the Coalition has been linked to a strong campaigning network: in addition to its county council funding the Coalition is also supported financially by a district council whose leader had been both a trade union activist and a member of a council which had rebelled against government legislation in the early 1970s. A local MP had also been active nationally on disability rights issues. Within this tradition, council support for the Coalition was seen as part of the wider struggle for civil rights for all citizens, properly placed within the mainstream political process:

> **"There is no doubt that it had to be politicised ... I mean it is disabled people within disabled organisations that know what being disabled is about and can fight through the political machinery for civil rights ... that can only be done by people that, miners get coal ... if somebody tells me they know what it is like working underground and they've never been underground I would call them a liar, they don't ... so people with disabilities who are running these sorts of organisations**

are the ones we accept know about these things, and it had to be brought into the political arena... (Leader, district council)

Within the NHS, however, the group's profile was rather different. The Coalition and the CIL have been seen as legitimate stakeholders whose views should be taken into account and balanced with all the other stakeholders and interest groups. While the NHS (manager) respondents stated a commitment to social models of disability, they also recognised that clinicans did not necessarily share these views:

"There is still tension between the social and the medical models of disability. There are still medics up at — hospital who I think do not agree with the whole approach of the young physically disabled strategy. Their view is that they could do more for disabled people in terms of rehabilitation etc, if they had them within their care, within the hospital. So I mean again, they didn't accept just user evaluation as being valid for looking at disability services ... there is always the two camps who are trying to increase the resources that they have and increase their share of the service which is being offered." (Purchaser, NHS)

From the perspective reported here the expert knowledge deriving from personal experience of disablement was not seen as a valid basis from which to reach decisions about the nature of services.

One NHS purchaser described the Coalition's early pioneering role:

"I think actually they were the first instance in which service users actually started to influence our policy as a health authority, back in the mid-1980s ... through the advocacy and they thrust themselves on us."

There were thus two main characterisations of the Coalition and the CIL: political actor/movement/force for change linked to local government, and legitimate stakeholder/consumer linked with the NHS. Both reflect the significant impact which the coalition and the CIL have made on the local health/social care scene. Although not accepted by all clinicians, the formal recognition of their specialist knowledge legitimates the position of both groups within the local 'apparatus of accountability' for services provided to disabled people and, more widely within an equal opportunities framework, to citizens as a whole. But for reasons sketched below, this influence and impact has begun to wane.

Many officials told us they believed the ascendancy of the Coalition originated with the activities of one of the organisation's founder members who also served as a county councillor. In addition, because it adopted a formal system of electing its ruling council, the Coalition became seen as a part of the operation of local representative democracy.

> **"Yes, that is certainly how it has been regarded in the Labour Group and especially at a time when it had a voice in, in a sense right in the middle of it when — was very visible there in his wheelchair, and a good advocate for it." (Leader, district council)**

Simultaneous with this type of influence there was a favourable political climate in which commitments were made by the then ruling Labour council leadership to supporting oppressed groups:

> **"But there has been a change in leadership too in the last three or four years. I guess I was the last one of the old leadership, ... until they removed me this year. Inevitably it brings a change in the way the group looks at things, but I don't think that's what has driven the cuts to CIL, although certainly CIL enjoyed really top level support from him [the county council leader] at that time, he saw it as a way of helping people he saw as oppressed, he felt very strongly about discrimination in all its forms..." (County councillor, now member of the CIL management committee)**

With the Coalition active from 1982 and the CIL from 1985, support from the county council had grown to a combined grant of almost half a million pounds (£448,000 of which £400,000 was for the CIL). Deep cuts were imposed in 1990, since when funding has shrunk progressively to present levels, with payment to the CIL down to around £152,000. This resulted in the loss of staff from both organisations and consequently a certain loss of influence over officials and ability to participate at many levels of service planning.

> **"Their grant funding was affected. They employed several people and now those are very, very few. So they've got less time to come out into the wider world and talk to people**

> like us. So we are now dependent on the access groups
> which are mainly volunteers. They used to have linkworkers
> attached to say two or three access groups, but they are not
> employed any more. They've got a sort of central organisation
> at — is it? I think it is, so the links even between them and
> the access groups have become a bit more tenuous. And
> probably as a result of that, I wouldn't say necessarily but –
> it may be just coincidental but I suspect because of that –
> one or two of the access groups have collapsed or lost
> interest..." (Officer, National Park)

The causes of the funding cuts have been the subject of much speculation.
Many officials were quick to refer to the 'official' reason – that is, rate or
community charge capping – while hinting at possible unofficial reasons.
These reflect the perceptions of the Coalition members interviewed. A
common unofficial reason concerned the Coalition's and the CIL's
propensity to 'rock the boat', that is, to be openly critical of county
council services while at the same time enjoying large-scale funding.

> "I mean historically there have been some difficult experiences
> and I think there was a legacy of 'CIL disapprove of us' type
> of thing. It was about trying to get people working together
> rather than them standing off each other ... one or two
> training events this sort of thing where strong views were
> expressed which people objected to. Well I suppose it was
> justified by CIL as that is what we are going to do, talk
> plainly about what we feel. But they clearly were seen as
> insensitive and narrow by others ... yes, there was a bit of a
> rift there..." (Manager, area social services)

Additionally, a growing problem was emerging about the relationship
between the Coalition, seen primarily as the campaigning arm, and the
CIL, funded as a major provider of services with a management
committee with 50% county council membership. With the CIL seen
as a provider in the 'new world' of contracting, county hall was seeking
greater control over both its expenditure within the CIL and the services
provided by it. This resulted in a more prescriptive attitude towards
what were then service agreements between the CIL and the county
council. In an increasingly market-oriented climate service providers
come under particular pressure not to engage overtly in 'politics', and if
those providers should be closely linked with campaigning they run the

risk of being marginalised. In contrast, the contracting process, involving the drawing up of specifications for services by the county council's legal department, is considered to be apolitical and 'objective'. The socially constructed nature of specifications and contracts is obscured by their official, quasi-legal language and framework.

> **"Well CIL was doing this campaigning stuff and it lost a lot of money as a result. Not just as a result, there were other things. [The Coalition] runs on much less resources. It is funded as an organisation which is representing, its campaigning is understood and it is accepted that it is a campaigning operation, and its funders are obviously happy with that. I mean when I'm talking about shouting the odds there is no purpose in just sort of saying everything is terrible. There are ways of making your point without terminally pissing off your funders." (Purchaser, NHS)**

These unofficial reasons for funding cuts were interrelated and were fairly widely alluded to by respondents. Interestingly one NHS official, more distanced from the controversy over the imposition of the local government cuts, mentioned allegations about 'financial irregularities' against the then CIL management which were made early in 1990. What part these allegations, which were never publicly resolved, played in the decision just five months later to withdraw £100,000 in funding is unclear. Coming on top of perceptions that the organisation was rocking the boat and failing to behave like a provider, by continuing to play an active part in disability politics, this financial story was very bad publicity for the CIL at a time when charge capping was being implemented and the county council was looking for cuts. This period seems to mark the height of the influence of both the Coalition and the CIL, following which there was a decline in activity.

The confusion over the relationship between the Coalition and the CIL was frequently referred to by officials. This issue seemed to spring from inherent contradictions, rather like the theory behind the NHS internal market. In theory the purchaser/provider division of labour appears workable – the Coalition would concentrate on campaigning and the CIL (now a registered charity) would concentrate on providing. In practice officials believed this was not working. Many Coalition activists were also employed by, or were part of, the CIL management. The *movement*, the Coalition, could not simply disengage from the *medium*, the CIL. If the CIL was established to be the realisation of the philosophy of integrated living for disabled people, it could not suddenly become a value-free agency. Service provision cannot take place in isolation from the politics of disability and it appeared that this was never the intention when the CIL was first established, as some officials recognised:

> "But that's how I see [the Coalition] and CIL. CIL was a sort of dream that this was the actual functional arm of those beliefs, that [the Coalition] was a bringing together of people to formulate a philosophy and ideas and CIL was one of the means of delivering it." (County councillor, CIL management committee)

The development of service agreements between the county and the CIL created a further dilemma. On one hand, the council was being faced with increasing demands to give account of the content of services it purchased with public money. On the other, the CIL believed it should be able to develop new types of service with that funding. The council's accountability (in the financial sense) to its wider constituents began to place constraints upon user group self-determination.

This political confusion came under sharp focus in the contracting process. With the implementation of community care reforms, the CIL became increasingly associated with the private/independent sector and ironically, therefore, as part of the draining away of county council powers.

> "... the desire of this [Conservative] government to see more things through community care put out to the private sector and voluntary sector and whether we like that or not in [county] social services, we've had to do a lot of that and it puts CIL firmly in that sector. But if you are putting things out like that then you have to have confidence in the fact that those organisations are well managed and run and will do a better job..." (County councillor, CIL management committee)

The following incident (which took place after interviews with Coalition members had been completed) illustrates this. In 1995 the CIL submitted a tender to provide technical aids services to the county council, but failed to win the contract. Politically the climate was very difficult:

> "The technical aids contract had to go out and CIL were one of the bidders, but they didn't get it. And there was a lot of

lobbying went on about that and a lot of discussion and a lot of difficulties." (as above)

The CIL's tender reflected its philosophy. Rather than tender for the provision of lists of equipment, specific pieces of hardware, their bid for what was seen by the purchaser as a discrete service centred more on individual assessment of needs and so was more open-ended. In this way the CIL was tendering to provide a hitherto very prescribed service, partly in order to change the way that service was provided. Setting aside the claim by some officials that the CIL's form of provision would have been more expensive, this was not the way that tendering had traditionally been carried out. It opened up, in the words of the officer involved, an "*inherent conflict*" between the users' philosophy and the assumptions behind contracting.

> **"Many of their comments at the management committee were around the need to change the nature of the contract had they won it ... I'm sure that would have been a serious problem to sort that out because the contract was very much drawn up by people in our solicitors' and central purchasing department, and although we are not hardly expert at it, it was to the best of the authority's knowledge, drawn up in a fairly tight, clear way... Ultimately although we have a lot of items, we would want to give individuals every chance to say what best suited them and try to respond to that. I mean ultimately [the Coalition] and CIL's position would be they don't agree with lists of equipment anyway, full stop, we should start from just looking at that person's needs and what is going to meet that need. I respect that view and in an ideal world that would be the way things are, but the legislative and financial pressures around the local authority do build in this problem all the time." (Development officer, social services)**

Ironically, while the contracting process allowed the CIL to enter the market, potentially increasing its sphere of influence, it appeared that prescriptiveness in service specifications played a part in preventing it from winning contracts. While timing of interviews meant that this particular incident was not discussed by Coalition interviewees, more general comments about a reluctance to engage with systems not consistent with their philosophy would anticipate a similar conclusion.

User groups, legitimacy and consumerism

Virtually all respondents agreed that the existence of groups such as the Coalition and the CIL helped to make services more accountable in the democratic sense. If services are seen to be accountable, then they are legitimised, along with the officials who still largely plan and purchase them. The Coalition has been the spearhead of user involvement in the county, but it is now in the position of witnessing the recognition/ promotion of other user groups as legitimate actors by officials. Rather than take account primarily of the Coalition, officials were attempting to build relationships with other organisations. Having accepted user involvement as *policy* (ie government-driven consumerism), officials were wary of potential dominance by one group. This conflicted with the Coalition's portrayal of itself as democratically representative of disabled people in the county. In the 'halcyon days' described above this representative role was less problematic (in the sense that the county council took a political decision to recognise the Coalition as a representative body). But in the culture of contracting, the actor-network has become drawn more widely. The tendering process engenders pluralist notions about servicing consumers or specific client groups; it does not promote representative democracy. The relationship between tendering/contracting in community care and service innovation is problematic. From our initial discussions about the technical aids contract, it seemed that the process, as then constructed, militated against innovation.

The decision not to award the contract for technical/home aids to the CIL was defended, on grounds of cost/value for money. In addition, when lobbied by the Coalition, officials who had built wider networks could also defend other decisions on the grounds of having to consult with a variety of specific user groups and individual users (rather than one prominent and articulate group), in order to promote diversity of response:

> "I think one of the difficulties that does emerge is that, it's the need to be aware that, for example, [the Coalition] is a highly politicised group, and understand the issues behind that politicisation. And almost the needs and wishes of other service users who are actually not politicised and have a very different perspective of what they want from us. So there is a hard balance between individuals who are politicised or groups who are politicised – it is not just [the Coalition] – it

is other groups that are to varying degrees, and other service users who haven't been reached by that activity..." (Planning officer, social services)

From the Coalition perspective, they have found themselves forced to play by the rules of a game which they have had no part in constructing and which they apparently cannot win – in spite of the rhetoric of responsiveness and participation. They share a wish to increase the legitimacy of State services, offering both a resource of expert knowledge, and a mechanism of accountability based in liberal democratic traditions. But ultimately, the imbalance of power has meant it has been possible for them to be squeezed out – except in those instances where it is in the interests of officials to include them.

Strategic userism – the user card

As we noted in Chapter 3 when discussing responses to the mental health group, some officials explicitly discussed 'playing the user card'. The search for diversity and plurality of consultee/input can sometimes stray into a more strategic activity of utilising user need or preference to promote the sectional or personal interests of officials. Purchasers and providers of health and social care, operating under the conflicting demands of both ensuring high quality and extracting value for money, must reach decisions after a process of negotiation between the two. One of the most important allies to have in the negotiation process is the user. This is partly because having the users on board strengthens the official's political position and partly because of issues to do with legitimacy mentioned above. Depending on the history of the situation, the alliance formed can be a partnership of equals, or it can amount to exploitation:

"I think as professionals, this is what I feel happens: that we make a decision that that is what we want to happen, and then we find users who want that to happen to support it. And it is really difficult to know if that is what everybody wants because you only get one or two with the energy because basically, it is very difficult to find the energy to come forward and plan." (Head of rehabilitation services, NHS Trust)

Another manifestation of 'playing the user card' is where the user groups can find themselves employed to help the officials fulfil requirements to consult and to be seen to be consulting. One voluntary sector provider working with an organisation providing support to carers told us she felt this was rather a cynical exercise:

> "I think it is all this, you know, saying they were actually consulting people and that they were funding these organisations. They wanted the innovative approach to things, people coming up with all these ideas..." (Coordinator, Crossroads)

Maintaining a close working relationship with an active user group can have unforeseen or indirect benefits for certain types of officials. We found an interesting example where the Coalition's lobbying actually materially benefited a major care provider in the county other than the CIL. As we have seen, lobbying by the Coalition on behalf of the CIL is increasingly problematic. The Coalition successfully lobbied on behalf of a number of users against a (purchaser) decision to switch to a cheaper provider. In this case the interests of the users were aligned with those of carers.

> "We've been quite involved with them [the Coalition and CIL] because we've had some problems with spot purchasing in — where social services have come along and said, 'Well, I'm sorry, you are too expensive now'. We can contract with a private agency. The carers have got very upset, it has been handled in a very insensitive way. The carers have got very upset about this and have contacted CIL. What I've tried to do is, I don't like to take over from people but I like to provide them with the information that if they are able to they can do it themselves. They contacted CIL and the Coalition intervened as well and fought the case for the carer, and really for Crossroads, because we're still in there ... we are not a campaigning organisation obviously. Indirectly it did us a lot of good... That was a major thing that they did because they took it up to county level. They wouldn't let go until ... they saw the whole lot through and I've got to say without the backing of CIL or, I mean the Coalition were involved as well on that one, things wouldn't have happened. They listened, county listened to what they'd got to say. I mean I believe it was a test case really. I think they have to

**look and be very careful you know with what they are doing
now." (Coordinator, Crossroads)**

In its campaigning role, the Coalition was able to pursue the issue further
than the provider here, resulting in the formation of an unexpected
alliance which both organisations could utilise in the future. (Unexpected
because Crossroads is principally a carers' organisation, serving a
constituency with sometimes conflicting interests from that of disabled
people/users.) Ironically the Coalition's lobbying for the retention of
particular carers (to the benefit of another provider) would not be open
to accusations of conflict of interest, such as it would if it was lobbying
for CIL.

Conclusion

There is evidence in this case study of both disabled people and officials
being forced into positions with which neither are entirely happy because
of ideologically driven structural changes in health and social care systems.
In the early to mid-1980s disabled activists and Labour politicians shared
a political analysis and understanding of the value of collective action to
resist oppression. The representative structure of the Coalition was
familiar to politicians used to negotiating with trade unions and a
combination of cooperation and opposition was sustainable within a
relationship which was seen to be beneficial to both parties who were
equally committed to the public provision of welfare.

However, as the local authority came under pressure from central
government, and as public provision of services was increasingly being
undermined by a government committed to the market, both the
Coalition and the local authority found their roles being redefined. For
the Coalition this meant learning the language of consumerism and,
albeit reluctantly, adopting strategies consistent with the purchaser/
provider split and which reflected financial transactions as a means of
control (see Chapter 5). The local authority, and more particularly the
health authority, came to regard the Coalition as one among a number
of stakeholder interest groups. In this position, and as potential
contractors to provide services, the Coalition and its 'provider arm' (the
CIL) were not to be 'privileged' as having any greater legitimacy or
representative role than any other voluntary or user organisation.

As the research was concluding, discussions were underway about
the future relationship between the Coalition and the CIL as well as
between the Coalition, the CIL and the county council. Such debates

reflect much wider shifts that are taking place as a new Labour government seeks a 'third way' between state and market in welfare provision.

•

FIVE

Consumers and citizens

Our earlier analysis of the policy context considered the very different meanings being ascribed to 'user involvement'. Certain of the tensions within that start to become evident in the case studies of the two groups we have described. In Chapter 1 we also highlighted the importance of distinguishing the roles of 'consumer' and 'citizen' when considering changes in the nature of relationships between the state and those who use public services. Having looked in some detail at two examples of user self-organisation and the response of public service officials to this, we can reflect on what this can contribute to our understanding of the role of user self-organisation in empowering people as consumers, and in enabling excluded people to become 'active citizens'.

Consumers and consumerism

User activists were very aware of the consumerist rhetoric which was enveloping health and social care services during the later part of the 1980s and into the 1990s. They also acknowledged the role this had played in creating an environment in which it was hard for officials to dismiss user views:

> "After that period of prior work, the establishment of the Coalition formation was against a background of acceptance by the authority that a consumer voice was a progressive step for the authority to take and that they should help it by funding it."

> "I think they want our opinions more than they used to do ... That's the current climate isn't it, user involvement."

However, while the language of consumerism had been well learnt by many of those active in the groups we studied, not all were entirely comfortable with it.

The attack on public service bureaucracies which came from the Conservative government of the 1980s and 1990s was based, in part, in a belief that producer interests had become too powerful and needed to be curbed (Harrison, 1991). One way of doing this was to introduce competition between providers. Another was to separate out responsibilities for determining what services were needed (purchasing or commissioning) from the direct provision of services. While the former should continue to be the responsibility of public authorities (in this context local government and health authorities), the provision of services should be carried out by a range of different provider agencies, including those operating in the commercial, voluntary and public sectors. This would ensure that those who needed to use services – consumers – would be able to exercise choice over which services they used and thus producers would be encouraged to increase the responsiveness of their services in order to attract consumers and stay in business. All this was based on a belief that public services could and should behave like private services. But the purchaser/provider splits in neither health nor social services provided direct consumer choice. They created 'quasi-markets' in which an agent (in the case of health services first the health authority and then GP fundholders) purchased on behalf of the consumer. Hence some might argue that the official injunctions to officials about being user responsive (such as the exhortation to health authorities to become 'champions of the people' in their purchasing strategies; NHSME, 1992) were necessary in order credibly to retain the rhetoric of choice which was introduced without any method for implementation. What we need to focus on here is the hegemony of the notion of 'choice' within this analysis.

Choice is the key metaphor of consumerism. The assumption is that those who use welfare services wish to make choices, that choices are possible, that it is a route to want and need satisfaction and inherently empowering. Choices are made by individual consumers determining their own needs and pursuing their individual self-interests. It is an essentially private action, with no sense that individual choices will have an impact on wider collective purposes or interests, nor that individuals should take account of those when making choices. If choice is to be a reality then there must be multiple sources of services from which to choose, and those services must be recognisably different.

Effective consumers are those who obtain information about available options, compare this with their knowledge and understanding of their own circumstances and needs, then choose which of the options on offer will best meet their needs. If they have problems they will complain and seek redress. If the situation is not resolved they may go elsewhere. Consumerist strategies seek to enable people to become more effective consumers by maximising these conditions. The sum total of individual actions is expected to influence the way in which producers behave, but consumer organisations also exist to represent the collective interests of individuals in their consumer role and act to counterbalance the power of producer interests (including organisations such as local authorities and professional bodies).

The concept of consumer choice was attractive to the Conservative government because it represented a constraint on the power of professionals who were seen as self-serving (not unlike trade unions). It offered similar attractions for those who had experienced substantial powerlessness in their relationships with welfare professionals and managers. The concept represents a rejection of the notion that people have to accept what they are given and accept the better judgement of producers about what is best for them. In Keat et al's (1994) terms, it emphasises the 'authority' of those who use services to determine their own needs and how they should be met. If it is accepted that people should be able to choose what music they listen to, what clothes they wear and what religious beliefs they hold, or indeed, if they hold any, why then should they not choose when and how they should receive medical treatment, from whom they should receive personal support, and whether they should attend day care?

Barnes and Prior (1995) have argued that there are many circumstances in which people use public services in which 'choice' may not be experienced as empowering, and, in some instances, may create a situation of risk and uncertainty which can be disempowering. They question whether it is choice per se that is valued, or getting what you want. While the experience of 'shopping around' can be an enjoyable one for some people in some circumstances, it does involve the expenditure of energies which may be in short supply. If people were able to influence and control how they receive services, would the opportunity to choose between them be so significant?

Nevertheless, past experiences of the absence of choice in the use of health and social care services meant that the consumerist rhetoric of the Thatcher years struck many chords for groups and individuals seeking to increase their control over welfare services which had become self-serving and unresponsive. Service brokerage, advocacy and the campaign for direct payments to enable users to purchase services directly without professional mediation all aim to increase both the opportunities and capacity for exercising choice in how and what services are to be received. In some instances that aim is expressed as a value in its own right. But often it is a means to exercising choice over how to live life as a whole.

Choosing to receive personal care support rather than spend two hours washing and dressing is a means of enabling someone to follow an education course or hold down a job, not a route to dependence.

In our analysis of user interviews we highlighted three key aspects of their responses to consumerism:

- what activists were saying about opportunities to exercise or extend the choices available to them as users of services;
- how they saw opportunities for improving the responsiveness of services; and
- 'market development' – the extent to which they were seeking to promote or contribute to the development of new or alternative forms of services which would enable users to 'shop around'.

The discourse of choice was prominent in interviews with activists in the groups studied. However, there were differences between these two groups in the extent to which explicitly consumerist strategies were seen as a route to empowerment. It is also important to consider what disabled people and the mental health user activists were saying about the focus of the 'choices' they were seeking.

User groups and consumerism

The mental health user group

The mental health user group's objectives in relation to choice were demonstrated in three ways. First, they sought to ensure people are provided with information to enable them to exercise choice on their own behalf. In particular, and in common with priorities which are widespread among users of mental health services, they were working to ensure that patients are given information about different forms of medication, their purpose and likely side effects. This is intended to enable people to be more assertive in expressing their wishes about treatment. It is an objective of individual advocacy in cases where the individuals themselves may not at the time be strong enough to express their own wishes.

Can ensuring that people are better informed about medical treatment be equated with the crafting of more effective consumers? 'Informed consent' is a right which can only be overridden in controlled circumstances even for those detained under the Mental Health Act. More generally medical treatment given without the consent of the recipient is unlawful except in cases of dire emergency. In this context, an objective of ensuring that people are better informed about medical treatment is better understood as a citizenship right (see below) than as part of a consumerist strategy. Closely related to this is the objective of ensuring that there is a variety of treatment options available to those who come into contact with mental health services. Information per se is not sufficient if psychotherapy and other forms of non-pharmaceutical treatment are unavailable unless bought privately. The group had pushed for the development of alternative forms of therapy (such as aromatherapy) to provide a wider range of options among which people can choose. But the overall objective was to ensure that people do not have to choose between providers in order to be able to choose between treatments or other interventions.

Enabling users to become consumers through purchasing services directly on their own behalf was not a priority of members of this group. It was included within the list of objectives of only one interviewee. Interviews were being conducted at a time when campaigning for direct payments was developing within the disability movement. However, responses of activists within the mental health group indicated that this was not an issue which had featured within their discussions. While there is a private market in psychiatry, psychotherapy and other forms of counselling and therapy (as there is in medicine generally) the cost of such services is beyond the means of the majority of those who experience mental health problems. When it is a struggle to ensure you receive benefit entitlements and can find somewhere decent to live, the option of shopping around for a private therapist is unlikely to be a priority.

At a collective level, the group's involvement in strategic decision making can be seen as having the objective of ensuring that people are not left without any option in relation to the way in which services are structured, or the type of services that are available. People exercise choice by means of selecting which service to enter, and exiting from services they don't like. The feasibility of this is severely constrained in relation to mental health services. Not only can people be forced to enter services (in the context of compulsory hospital admissions), but for the majority of people with mental health problems the option of shopping around is unrealistic because of poverty – and at times of great emotional distress motivation to obtain information about a range of services and select between them is low. One activist was clear that the exercise of choice by means of exit would represent a failure to achieve their objectives. For example, a failure to prevent the merging of geographical sectors through which services in the city were organised, in the face of opposition from users, was considered to have left people with 'exit' as their only option in terms of the exercise of choice:

> **"It puts us in a position of either having to pursue a line that we know we're not going to get any change by refusing to participate in the centre, or encouraging people to make the best of a bad job, basically. And I think that's absolutely diabolical because had they really consulted people they would never have made the proposal to reduce the number of sector teams in the first place."**

The question of service responsiveness is closely linked to that of choice. The notion of a responsive service can refer to apparently mundane matters: such as a situation in which a shortage of towels available on wards meant that people were using sheets to dry themselves; or to the importance of flexibility in services in order to take account of the impact which mental ill health may have on people's ability to adhere to strict timetables (this example referred to training courses intended to enable people to develop skills such as carpentry, brickwork and painting and decorating). Responsiveness also relates to accessibility, and 24-hour access to crisis services was something this group had been seeking to achieve.

Market development can include developing the range of providers within the voluntary as well as the private sector. Although user movements have developed in part in distinction from voluntary organisations *for* rather than *of* disabled people, constitutionally many would be located as part of the voluntary sector. The option of entering the market as service providers is one that is open to them and one of the other mental health groups in this study had started and continued as the provider of a service which was deliberately intended to offer an alternative to day services provided by statutory health and social care agencies. However, the group considered here does not see itself as being in the business of market development on its own behalf. Apart from the caravan purchased to enable people to take holidays, the only 'services' it provides are information and advocacy services. Through Ecoworks, the environmental work project, work can be undertaken on contract to other agencies, but these are not services which are in competition with statutory mental health services. The suggestion that the group should develop and run a 24-hour crisis service was being treated very cautiously because of the acknowledged tension between service provision and acting as advocates on behalf of service users.

The disabled people's Coalition

All those we interviewed believed that the Coalition should aim to improve the choice available to disabled people over which services they are able to use. Three people chose this as one of their three priority aims. Improvement in the access of existing services was chosen as an aim by eight interviewees. One interviewee described 'Choice and control' as the guiding principle behind the Coalition.

However, the motivation to develop the CIL was less about providing individual disabled people with a choice over which service to use, than a demonstration of the benefits of services based on alternative models of disability. Increasing choice was not seen necessarily as involving the Coalition or indeed the CIL in establishing services in competition to those provided by traditional service providers, and the CIL was always conceived as a joint venture with the local authority. However, since the data collection was completed the CIL has been involved in competing for contracts to provide services. This is something the group is not entirely happy about and which is in large part a response to the reduction in core funding for the group and the extension of contracting as the mechanism through which services can be provided from the independent sector.

The 'choices' being sought through the establishment of the CIL were primarily opportunities for disabled people to choose how to live their lives, rather than which service to turn to for help. One example of this is the peer counselling service being provided through the CIL. This service enables individuals to discuss their situation with a disabled Coalition member prior to assessment and decisions being made concerning needs by the service providers:

> **"Having somebody you can talk to about possibilities and help build confidence, you can introduce the idea that these things are manageable. And not only that, that you can make a better job of managing it yourself than anybody else is going to do it for you."**

For one woman that we interviewed it was important:

> **"... to maintain disabled people in their own homes, and to make resources available to that end, so that the Coalition can actually support disabled people and help them to make decisions, to widen their choices and help them to make**

decisions about their lives. And to keep them out of
institutional care."

In this context 'choice' clearly refers to life choices rather than shopping
around between services. The Coalition has consequently lobbied and
written papers to support this aim and to encourage service providers
to think in this way. If, according to one interviewee, the system worked
well:

"... disabled people in addressing services would be able to
define what services are needed and expect service providers
to identify and train and manage the technicians to support
that."

The objective of ensuring control over life choices had led many disabled
people to conclude that this was best achieved through enabling the
direct purchase of support services. Eight of the people that we
interviewed identified enabling disabled people to purchase their own
services directly as an aim of the Coalition and four chose this as a
priority. One interviewee saw this as a way of disabled people taking
control and of removing the fear of service withdrawal if complaints or
comments were made to service providers. Seven of the people that we
interviewed believed that enabling disabled people to become their
own care managers was an objective of the Coalition and five people
chose this as a priority.

"More and more disabled people by being empowered and
listening to other disabled people and actually demanding
choices and control, then that's starting to come about and
the more and more disabled people who believe that and
actually start putting that into practice then, it's taking back
what is ultimately their money to buy back some of the
services they want."

But even this consumerist development was seen as something best
pursued by means of cooperation among disabled people, rather than
through individual disabled people competing with each other by, for
example, offering more attractive terms and conditions in order to attract
the 'best' care assistants. It has been made possible by the collective
organisation of disabled people, rather than by the assertive individualism
of competing consumers.

Another interviewee talked of the increase in choice that was required concerning, for example, wheelchair provision. She talked of her own personal difficulty with regard to a power wheelchair that she requires; she can be provided with either an indoor power chair or an outdoor power chair but not one that is suitable for both indoor and outdoor use. She could buy an expensive suitable wheelchair herself if she had the money. This example illustrates potential differences in the comparative priorities attached by members of the two groups to the opportunity to purchase services directly. A wheelchair can be seen as a commodity for which it is possible to shop around in order to find the type which is best suited to a particular person. Having bought it, it will need maintenance and occasional repairs, but the transaction is largely completed at the time of purchase. This involves a different relationship between consumer and 'product' from that involved in the purchase of, for example, counselling. In that case the transaction is emergent and on-going and it is through that continuing transaction that the service is provided. In economists' terms, counselling is an 'experience good' which can only be known in the process of use – it cannot be tried out to see if it fits before buying.

There was clearly ambivalence among some Coalition activists about an emphasis on individualistic solutions to the experiences of disabled people. While the responses of interviewees indicate a strong commitment to influence and control over the services they need in order to enable them to live their lives as they want, their preferred way of achieving this is through influencing and being part of the management of services provided from within public sector organisations, rather than developing a market in services. The pressure on the CIL to seek to enter into contractual arrangements with the local authority with whom it had sought to work in partnership in the development and management of the CIL was causing tensions within the Coalition. These are continuing through internal reviews of the relationship between the two arms of the local movement.

Thus while user groups are seeking more information to enable people to exercise more choice from a wider range of services, and while some are seeking to control the services they receive by making purchases unmediated by professional assessment, this is primarily within the context of public sector services, or being made possible by the collective organisation of disabled people and those with mental health problems. Cooperation rather than competition was seen as the force for empowerment in relation to the provision of more responsive services. Whether this will remain the case following the development of direct payments schemes is perhaps uncertain. The role of disabled people's organisations in supporting those opting for direct purchase may well increase, but it remains to be seen whether an extension of such roles under contract to local authorities will limit the broader campaigning objective of disabled people's organisations. It is also by no means clear that mental health user groups will see the extension of direct payments as the preferred strategy for empowering users of mental health services.

One crucial limitation of the concept of consumerism for understanding the way in which user groups seek the empowerment of disabled people and those with mental health problems is that it refers solely to the relationship between users and services. User groups have objectives beyond those of exerting influence over health and social care services and, as we have seen, the choices they are seeking are not only or primarily choices concerning welfare services. For this reason if for no other, it is inadequate to view consumerist tactics as a route towards empowerment and we also need to consider how an analysis based in notions of citizenship can contribute to an understanding of the projects in which user groups are engaged.

User groups and citizenship

Citizenship refers to the relationship between individuals and the State, or the political community of which they are members. There are three key aspects of that relationship which are of particular significance in this context.

First, services provided by or through the State should be *accountable* to citizens, that is, those responsible for taking decisions about the nature of services, the allocation of resources to them, the policies and criteria for access to them, should both give account of their decisions and the reasons for taking them, and be able to be held to account by citizens for those decisions (Ranson and Stewart, 1994).

Second, membership of a political community confers certain *rights* on citizens:

- legal or civil rights enable the individual to participate freely in the life of the community; own property; enter into contracts; engage in religious practice or other forms of collective association;
- political rights entitle the citizen to participate in the government of the community by voting, standing for election etc;
- social and economic rights are less clearly defined but are intended to enable the individual to participate in the general well-being of

the community and include rights to health care, education, welfare (Marshall, 1950; Plant, 1992).

There is no constitutional statement about inalienable rights in the UK and all these rights have been subject to negotiation and conflict and are open to change. The right to silence in criminal proceedings is one example. Many social rights have never been enshrined in statute and are thus often subject to decision making by gatekeepers. There is a duty on the NHS to provide services, rather than an individual right of citizens to receive health care. The assumption that an assessment of need under the 1990 NHS and Community Care Act would lead to the provision of services was successfully challenged by Gloucestershire County Council and even if needs have been agreed, receipt of services is often contingent on the availability of services rather than being there as of right.

Third, alongside 'rights' are placed 'obligations': if citizens have a right to receive welfare they also have an obligation to pay taxes if they meet the criteria. This raises the question of what citizens might be expected to 'do' – this is the issue which Prior, Stewart and Walsh (1995) address in their concern with 'the practice of citizenship'. They emphasise a practice of citizenship which is based on *interactive participation* in the political community in which citizens are active contributors to the process of collective decision making.

There are thus three themes which reflect different aspects of the relationship between users who are also citizens and services which are provided if not by the state, then as a result of statutory provisions: accountability of services to citizen users; the rights of citizen users to receive services which will enable general participation in the life of the community; and the active contribution that citizen users can make to determining the nature of services and of social life more generally.

The effective consumer and the active citizen are thus rather different and have different implications for the way in which people who use services may play an increasing part in their production. Once again we will consider how those active in these two groups saw the issue of citizenship in the context of their objectives and strategies.

Mental health, 'incapacity' and citizenship

Rights

For people with mental health problems the issue of citizenship rights has a particular significance because of the possibility that certain of these rights will be removed if they are compulsorily detained under the 1983 Mental Health Act. During the time we were conducting this study, the introduction of supervision registers intended to monitor the movements of certain discharged patients was a live issue. It had been the subject of discussion within the Patients' Council locally and the mental health group discussed here had also been involved in national discussions on the issue. There was also reference to the group's involvement in ensuring that people were represented at Mental Health Review Tribunals, and that people had the opportunity to exercise their right to complain through complaints procedures:

> **"One strand of the advocacy group (is) ... trying to get access to information and guiding people in knowing the system and knowing how to get the best out of the health services, how to appeal against sections of the Mental Health Act and all those sorts of things where perhaps ordinarily people would advocate for themselves, but in a period of crisis they need that bit extra support."**

Rights issues were also referred to in relation to welfare benefits where the regulations with regard to entitlements deriving from mental illness were considered to be unclear. The group had made some input to the campaign for anti-discrimination legislation, but this had not been a major focus of the group's activity. There were also expressions of disappointment that there was no indication that community care services would be made legal entitlements. Nevertheless one interviewee considered it important that legislation should be considered as a way of increasing public awareness and contributing to changing attitudes about both mental health and disability.

Other references to rights were not concerned with formal entitlements to services or benefits, but with notions of social justice. This included people's rights to have their voices heard and respected when they were expressing wishes *not* to receive certain forms of treatment (ECT for example), or *to* receive treatment – as in the case of the person refused Clozapine because of the cost; and the expectation that people discharged from hospital would be provided with some form of accommodation as a basic necessity for life in the community.

Accountability

Accountability can be exercised at very different levels. At an individual level it was considered to mean fair treatment, ensuring that patients know all their rights under the Mental Health Act and all the potential services which are available to them in the community. At a ward level, taking up patients' concerns about the quality of food was considered to be a means of holding managers to account:

> **"They are not perhaps big issues, or some are I think. We've tried to get improvements to the service and management are accountable because they have the money don't they?"**

At a broader level there was a view that managers needed to be made aware if they were spending money on services which were not producing benefits for their users. The group was considered to have an important role in this:

> **"I think it's very easy for professionals to write a really glowing document saying this is what we are providing, but if the end result is that it is not what is really happening, then they have to be made accountable for that particular statement and so one of the roles I think we play is to actually challenge the quality assurance issues, for instance, laid down in the contract between the mental health unit and the purchasing group of the health authority. And if they don't meet that then we will actually raise it both with the provider and say you're not meeting it and if we don't get any response we'll raise it with the purchaser and say, you know, what are you going to do about this?"**

As well as using the contracting system to hold both purchasers and providers to account, the group also confronts individual managers "putting them in the hot seat if you like", in order to get them to explain directly to users why they are not providing the service people want.

One interviewee talked of the issue of accountability in terms both of the need for public services to be publicly accountable, and for more direct accountability to be given to service users. He also noted that private meetings of the Trust Board got in the way of accountability:

"I think there's a general accountability but I think there's a very specific accountability to users of the service, particularly accountability if there's a history to redress that service users have had next to no involvement, no accountability, no choices over the last decade, so I think there's a particular duty to make it a very clear accountability now to service users."

He saw the mechanism through which such accountability could be exercised as residing in the Patients' Council:

"I think that is a good method of accountability and I think the Patients' Council works well because it does work on the principle that it's not one or two service users ... sitting on the edge of a meeting or a Trust Board or management meeting or whatever, it is managers, senior managers coming to meetings of service users to be accountable and really they have to account on the spot. They're not getting into delayed correspondence or anything..."

Participation

The notion of participation can itself be subdivided. First, user groups provide opportunities for people whose confidence has been undermined by mental distress to become involved within an organisation in which their experience is valued and in which they can grow in safety. Second, through such involvement, people may be empowered to participate more widely in the social and economic life of society. And third, user groups provide opportunities for people to exercise choice about whether to engage in services as either consumers or producers.

Examples were given of people who had been members of local groups supported by the city-wide group who were encouraged to become active participants and who now undertook key roles within the group. That active involvement had been a source of empowerment for members:

"It's given me a life and without it I wouldn't have dreamed of doing half the things I do now. It's given me confidence, assurance ... I get up now and speak at a conference quite happily. A few years ago I would have no more done that than fly!"

It was also considered by one interviewee to be a means through which people could explore and develop their understanding of what empowerment can mean. This can provide a route into broader community participation:

> **"For me the important thing in my bit of [the group] is to work at the end of empowerment which relates to employment, involvement in citizenship roles, leisure, education and training. I think it is important to stress because as I say, [the group] is broad and that's a healthy thing of it, the notion of empowerment and user involvement has gone way beyond a simple definition and I think the fact that [the group] is working at each of the different angles is good, it's a strength..."**

Empowerment through participation in a collective movement of people who are or have been users of mental health services can operate at a personal level through overcoming stigma, developing self-confidence and a sense of being valued. This can enable people to start to take control of their own lives. But that personal growth takes place within the context of the collective experience of the group as a whole:

> **"... also it's nice to think you've grown and been recognised, I mean I suppose that's a bit of self glory isn't it? But, I think you've achieved, you've managed to help people through these times and you have a look back and think, well, if we hadn't been there as a group, this wouldn't have got done."**

People are more able to assert their individual wishes because they know others are doing the same and they know the group is there to back them up. Empowerment can also come through demonstrating, to both professionals and other users, that users of mental health services are capable of participating in decision-making structures:

> **"One of the major roles that we play is actually to say, we are users, we can participate at this level, we can articulate, we can challenge, we can negotiate, we can write papers, we can do this, instead of [being] some bumbling idiot that doesn't know what they are doing."**

The employment of paid workers and volunteers who have themselves used mental health services is both a means and an end in itself. The individuals themselves develop skills from which both they and the group benefit, while also being enabled to participate as citizens through contributing their work to the group. Some subsequently go on to employment elsewhere:

> **"We've had about three or four young women that have started and we've had one young man here, he was both physically and mentally disabled and when I first met him, I thought never in my life are you going to get fit to get a job. He's working for the council full time!"**

In the case of those who are members of user groups supported by the city-wide group, supporting participation can require considerable input to motivate people, and a high level of organisation:

> **"The people at — once a week for the cooking, the minibus comes and fetches them now and takes them down there to the college, they like using the big kitchen. So you see, some can't even go on a bus without company, they've got to get into taxis and things, so we try to get them out more, so that's good fetching them down there."**

Enabling that wider participation also requires overcoming the discrimination which prevents people with mental health problems being considered as potential employees, or indeed people to live next to or to invite into your own home. One example of the problem was described by one interviewee:

> **"People are discharged into the community and what happens is that people are being put in the same area – so that you are getting groups of people with mental health problems clearly in one particular sector. This is not integration, it's a form of segregation and it shouldn't be happening."**

Mental Health Awareness Week is intended to break down barriers which get in the way of people with mental health problems participating within the local community. In addition to this, other smaller scale initiatives have been designed to overcome barriers to participation:

> **"One I can think of that instantly comes to mind is a ward**

> called — which is a long-term ward, long-stay ward, they're moving together and there's arrangements made that, at the end of September, the borough council are having a holiday and the whole of the ward is going to introduce themselves to people within the locality and say, 'Here we are. Tough, you've got us, but let's live side by side.'"

The ecological work projects developed under the umbrella of the group as a whole are focused on enabling people with mental health problems to participate as citizens in social and economic initiatives which are also considered to offer a model for small-scale local development which could enable the participation of other excluded groups:

> "There's also simultaneously this interest in the city council on these community empowerment issues. How do you help deprived areas become more assertively involved? There's potentially a block of people here who are interested in this, who can actually get some projects off the ground. So I think connecting into locality regeneration programmes is very exciting."

Disability rights and citizenship

> "If it was me speaking for the Coalition then perhaps even the Coalition itself would be more ... the emphasis would be on the idea of citizenship rather than consumerism."

Rights

The notion of rights was both implicit and explicit in many of the comments made by interviewees in the disabled people's Coalition. They referred to rights to services, the right to run their own affairs and the right to be treated with equality and respect: "It's rights and not charity, you don't want handouts"; "All we ask for is fair and what's reasonable in society. To give us a fair standard, a fair crack in life, that's all we're asking for. The same kind of issues that able-bodied people take for granted"; "We are part of the country, it's the government's responsibility to provide these things for us, not the charities to raise money."

Social rights involve access to public services in addition to 'welfare'. Most of the interviewees saw the role of the Coalition as improving disabled people's access to employment, leisure and recreational facilities and educational and training opportunities. For several people access to the built environment was an obvious first step to achieving this:

"Total access first and foremost for disabled people, because if you haven't got the access, it's no good applying for the job is it? And it's no good going to college or university if I've got a mountain of steps to go up."

In this context, the campaign for anti-discrimination legislation was an important focus for the Coalition at the time of interviews. All saw the achievement of such legislation as an aim for the Coalition and five people saw it as a major aim: "I can go into a pub and the landlord will be about to say, 'I don't have cripples in here'; we need protection in the law to prevent that sort of thing happening"; "We have got to get parliament to bring in legislation. That's what the crux is all about, to stop discrimination."

The Coalition was heavily involved in this campaign, working closely with MPs and the media, organising trips to London for demonstrations and lobbying and more general letter-writing and postcard campaigns. Non-members were involved as well.

For one interviewee the issue of anti-discrimination legislation opened up the profound questions of "where the responsibility of the State lays and how does the State and the individual interact and on what basis does it interact." Legislation of this type, he felt, might not be the most desirable outcome: "It carries with it always the possibility of the confrontational ethos, an attritional process rather than something else."

He looked towards an alternative lifestyle where participation "could be expressed in a much different way in the streets, villages, community involvement and everything else". This reflects a concept of citizenship as participation as well as rights and we consider this in more detail below.

Some spoke of the passage of legislation as the first step; the implementation of any Act was the test of the commitment of the government: "I don't think it will be the end, I think it will be the beginning."

Accountability

All those we interviewed believed that the Coalition should aim for an improvement in the accountability of services to those who use them and five chose this as a priority aim. The Coalition has representatives on service planning groups and local planning groups who are able to hold the service providers to account:

> **"It's so important that the powers that be, you know, they've got to let people know what they're doing, why they're doing it, and how they're doing it. You know, this closed door business is just not on."**

One interviewee remarked on how difficult this can be for officers of the authority:

> **"It raises, it seems, many issues as to how the officers of the authority deal with the questions that are raised. They are not used to being accountable to the member of an organisation, they are not used to being asked awkward questions, and so it is a very difficult environment."**

He went on to suggest that if direct experience of disability was accepted as being essential to service planning and provision then "The Coalition could become a formal part of the apparatus of accountability". At the present time "lip-service" was being paid to such a development.

Individual disabled people can find it difficult to hold service providers to account:

> **"Accountability – they had no way of actually complaining; they were scared to complain because the services might be pulled on them."**

One interviewee saw the relationship between users and service providers as paternalistic – an approach which does not sit easily with accountability. And another interviewee commented: "I think social services still feel that it is for them to say whether it has been a good service or not."

This interviewee saw the Coalition's role as "to encourage the providers to accept criticism" but also "to get disabled people more confident to challenge, to make the service providers accountable to them."

Participation

Participation on equal terms with able-bodied people is high on the agenda for the Coalition. When asked about the guiding principle behind the Coalition one interviewee said: "equality of participation, I think that's the guiding light we try to follow."

Interviewees spoke of members who had been able to get jobs, or to participate in leisure activities following their confidence-building involvement with the Coalition. The political character of the Coalition encourages a view of the importance of disabled people's participation in politics and in public bodies:

> "**Increasing the participation ... absolutely, yes. I mean there's a lot of disabled people who have a real contribution to make to local and national politics but in some instances it is not possible because again the environment's against us.**"

> "**More (disabled) women are having relationships ... getting married ... having children. So it is obvious to anybody that we need access to health care, we need access to schools, disabled parents need to be able to go on to Board of Governors and things like that to have a say in their child's education ... But we still can't get the message over to everybody because it is not part of policy, we can't get it into policy.**"

One interviewee defined the explicit guiding principle behind the Coalition as "Active citizenship" and defined this as follows:

> "**It's a necessary part of the historical process for each individual to be engaged in the society in which they live, essentially with a sense of individual and social self.**"

> "**It's sad that in a progressive country there is still segregated education and segregated transport, segregated day centres and everything else. We are still unable to accept people for what they are.**"

Conclusion

Officials who view user groups as just another self-interested stakeholder within a pluralist system of decision making about welfare services focus on their role in enabling people to become more effective consumers of services. There is benefit to providers in ensuring greater responsiveness to user needs since this will enhance their legitimacy and contribute to their survival within a (quasi-) market. There is also a genuine wish among many to ensure that services are more responsive, and an increasing willingness to recognise the knowledge and expertise of those for whom relationships with health and social care services can continue for many years.

However, to understand the role of such groups as equivalent solely to that of a consumer organisation is to lose sight of their significance in challenging the exclusion of disabled citizens from all aspects of social, economic, political and cultural life. Participation in groups can be a source of valued roles for people whose competence has been questioned and whose lives have been constrained by poverty and discrimination as well as by the effect of exclusionary social polices. Participation provides experience of the potential of collective action for social change as well as a forum in which personal experiences can be theorised and new knowledge developed. User groups contribute to action within civil society through which both welfare and government can be democratised.

SIX

Conclusion

Introduction

In Chapter 5 we sought to draw from our case study material some conclusions related to our conceptual themes of consumerism and citizenship. In this final chapter we draw together the main points which arise from the case studies in Chapters 3 and 4 as they apply to more practical issues. Where appropriate, reference is made to the more general findings of the larger study.

User views on the policy context: new management and community care

The aims of the two groups considered in some detail in this report (and indeed of the other four groups in our study) went beyond bringing about change in what were seen as inadequate, dependency-creating statutory services. Although changes in service planning and provision resulting from the 1990 Act had inevitably impinged on the groups and the way that they worked, they did not define the groups' purposes. Thus they also focused on the legacy of prejudice, discrimination, exclusion and disempowerment which disabled people and people with mental health problems experience in all areas of their life. In the case of Group One, this related to the stigmatising nature of mental health problems, while Group Five had a more far-reaching view, based on a social model of disability.

Neither group felt that their relationships with local statutory agencies were bad, but Group One reported a more positive relationship with the NHS than with local authorities and Group Five vice versa. Neither group (nor any of the others in the study) criticised the principle of community care, but were critical of what they saw as failure to resource its successful implementation. In particular, restrictions on local government finance had also affected the funding of user groups. Moreover, the purchaser/provider split had resulted in a proliferation of bodies that user groups may wish to influence, meaning that decisions had to be made about priorities. Concern was expressed that these organisational changes had led user groups to become more reactive rather than proactive.

User groups' objectives and strategies

Hirschman (1970) identified three broad models of the way in which actors might respond to dissatisfaction with an organisation: 'exit', 'voice' and 'loyalty'. The user groups in our study employed all of these, together with a fourth, to which we refer as 'rewriting the rules' (see below). It is evident that groups are prepared to adopt a variety of strategies in different circumstances. However, different strategies might conflict; for instance, campaigning might compromise the ability to enter into contracts to provide services.

Loyalty

Partnership and joint working were evident through the involvement of user groups in official forums; the examples that follow are drawn from all the groups in our study. Group One met with the district health authority to discuss the content of service contracts, while Group Two was involved in organising a regional conference held by the national Mental Health Task Force User Group. Members of Group Three had attended a stakeholders' conference and Group Four was represented on the Strategic Framework Group which is the service purchasing group in the area. Group Five had developed and subsequently managed a Centre for Integrated Living in partnership with the county council and Group Six was involved in task-based working groups (eg on transport) set up by the Joint Partnership Group. In addition, all the groups apart from Group Three were seeking to influence the content of service contracts placed elsewhere.

Exit

Only Group Three had a priority to provide an alternative to statutory services. Other groups did not consider themselves to be providing services set up in competition with the statutory sector. However, all provided information and advice services and two mental health groups were under contract to provide advocacy services. Through the Centre for Integrated Living, Group Five had also become involved in competing for service contracts. All three disability groups supported initiatives to enable disabled people to purchase their own services directly and two were involved in schemes to assist people to employ their own care assistants. Nevertheless, groups expressed little enthusiasm either for involvement in contracting as a way of achieving influence, or for the purchaser/provider split.

Voice

All but one of the groups aimed to exert influence over statutory services through the expression of 'voice' both inside and outside the system. (Group Three was pessimistic about the possibility of achieving change in mainstream services.) Voice could be expressed through individual advocacy, or through campaigning or lobbying. The voice to be heard was variously a consumer voice; the 'expert' voice; the voice that had never been listened to; a voice calling officials to account. The groups aimed to encourage and support people to find their voices, and to ensure they were listened to.

All the groups were to some extent involved in campaigning and politics, though only one of the three mental health groups saw itself primarily as a campaigning group. Campaigning involved using media and political contacts to achieve influence, as well as the collection of evidence to support their case (as in the 'Stress on Women' campaign led by MIND in which Group Two had a high profile). Interviewees in one group felt it would be difficult for them to take a definite stance on campaigning issues because of their commitment to the representation of different individual positions through advocacy. All the disabled people's groups used campaigning tactics including lobbying local and national politicians in support of anti-discrimination legislation; campaigning 'within the system'; using their positions in local planning forums and the like to pursue specific issues; and mounting local events to raise public awareness.

Those groups which were active campaigners also made use of the media to achieve influence. Group Two had a media adviser. Group Five had also had a high media profile at different times. Group One made use of local media in publicising Mental Health Awareness Week.

Rewriting the rules

A final set of strategies adopted by user groups can be seen as attempts to escape from present constraints by changing the assumptions upon which the present system operates: rewriting the rules, as it were. User groups sought not only practical changes, but changes in the way in which professionals and lay people think about disability and mental distress. These ideological objectives are assisted through the groups' involvement in research, training and theoretical work.

Four groups had been involved in formal training of practitioners, managers or both. All the groups undertook informal research through discussion with their members or contacts. Some had undertaken more specific research linked to individual campaigns. One was actively involved in contributing to the theoretical base of disability politics through publication and research. Another was involved not only in developing alternative understandings of mental distress, but giving practical expression to this through environmental employment schemes.

Most felt that their priorities were to influence health and social care services, but all had additional, broader aims, including improving employment, education and training opportunities; improving physical access; influencing public perception; encouraging participation in politics; seeking amendments to welfare legislation and specific rights to services; and achieving anti-discrimination legislation. Thus Group One was developing local action linking ideas about sustainable development to the creation of lifestyles protective of people's mental health. Group Five saw much of their work as representing disabled people not as dependants in need of care, but as citizens with rights to participate in society on equal terms with able-bodied people. Consequently they campaigned for resources to be invested in supporting the integration of disabled people into mainstream life and worked with architects, engineers, planners and designers.

Yet another approach to rewriting the rules was direct action, a tactic used by the radical end of the user movement. Groups seem to accept a 'division of labour' among their members; there is a recognition that people should make their own choice about such action. For some it can be an important way of experiencing a sense of power, while others feel physically vulnerable. While it did not figure as a prominent method for influence, it had been used in both planned and unplanned ways. Thus one group stormed a conference on sexuality and disabled people to which no disabled people had been invited; and there was a spontaneous 'take-over' by Group One of a meeting discussing plans for the reorganisation of mental health services.

Empowerment and autonomy

It is difficult to avoid the conclusion that the user groups in our study had achieved for themselves, and sometimes for those they sought to represent, a degree of influence that could not have been achieved by individuals. Yet the groups' influence remained fragile, for three (overlapping) reasons.

One reason is material. Groups were chronically unstable in terms of funding, even those, such as Group Five, which had once seemed in secure command of considerable resources, and most had experienced recent cuts. Several interviewees commented that this could affect the way that user groups operated – making them less outspoken or critical, or alternatively making them more politically active.

Another reason relates to the groups' human resources. There was a constant effort required to maintain an adequate level of activists. This was particularly difficult for mental health groups (where periods of illness could deplete the number of people available), but both Groups One and Five had an increasingly ageing active membership. (It may well be that this is a reflection of broader social change in respect of declining rates of participation in non-work organisations.) These problems also added to problems of credibility (see below); groups had good reasons for adopting the pragmatic approach to the question of group membership described in Chapters 3 and 4, but the inability to demonstrate a mass formal membership undoubtedly hampered their ability to be recognised as representative.

The third reason relates to the position of managers and professionals. It is certainly the case that government injunctions to listen to users have had some effect in changing officials' attitudes. Yet, as we have seen, the latter have retained the ability to adopt a tactical approach: to accept user groups, their activities and opinions when it suits local officials and to de-legitimise them in various ways when it does not. As long as managers' roles are seen as 'holding the ring' among a plurality of stakeholders (of whom organised users are only one) in statutory services, the opportunity for them to attend only selectively to user voices will remain.

Policy implications

If policy makers are genuinely committed to greater user involvement in the design, planning and delivery of services, then user *self*-organisation needs to be both encouraged and supported materially without being 'captured' by or incorporated into management. This implies not only that groups should be afforded some official status in the hierarchies of statutory organisations, but that the performance management systems applied to those organisations should include audits of responsiveness to them. Since the research was completed, the election of a new Labour government has created a different context within which relationships between statutory organisations and user groups will develop. Increasingly public agencies are being enjoined not only to develop partnerships with each other in order to deliver public policy objectives, but also to develop partnerships with community organisations. In our initial discussions with umbrella organisations at the start of this project they expressed considerable caution about the notion of 'partnership' because of the unequal power relationships involved. Thus we adopted the term 'joint working' rather than partnership to describe situations in which user groups felt their objectives might best be achieved by working within the system, rather than campaigning or direct action outside it. Whether or not relationships between user groups and health or local authorities might in future be described as relationships of partnership will depend not only on the preparedness of officials to recognise such groups as having a position which is different from that of other 'stakeholders', but also on whether user groups feel confident that their objectives can be met within the closer relationships implied by partnership.

Future enquiry

Our findings contribute to the understanding of how local governance is affected by bodies outside the formal organs of governance and we think that our findings suggest four areas for further work. First, there is clear scope for the in-depth exploration of the 'user as expert' and its implications for professional/managerial authority. As we noted in Chapter 1, a number of formal provisions have been made for national level user involvement in Research and Development and in the oversight of National Service Frameworks, and both these developments can be seen precisely as casting users in the role of experts, alongside other kinds of expert. The impact of these innovations needs to be monitored though, as we go to press, it has been reported that some consumer members of the group overseeing the creation of the National Service Framework for mental health services have resigned in protest at government insistence that compulsory treatment orders are non-negotiable (*Health Service Journal*, 12 November 1998, p 5).

Second, there is a need for methodological development of research working *with* user groups. Again, there are national attempts to encourage such working, both (as noted above) through the Standing Advisory Group on Consumer Involvement (in Research and Development) and through the formal requirements of some central programmes (such as *Health in Partnership*) for projects to include users. An overview project of the workings and outcome of such involvement would provide a valuable guide to future work.

Third, there are questions about how participation can be further developed, in some cases where no groups exist, perhaps by community development approaches. One possible vehicle for such development is the concept of the 'Health Action Zone', currently being implemented in a number of pilot sites throughout England. Although each local initiative is unique, all presuppose a more holistic and multi-agency approach than has been customary, and many require close liaison with user groups. All these initiatives are to be the subject of separate local evaluations, and of an overall national evaluation which will include a study of community development and public participation. This should offer useful lessons about community development and about the extent to which 'partnership' represents a genuine opportunity for user and community groups to be a part of the process by which rules are set, rather than occupying a reactive position.

Finally, there is a need for research to link the user/statutory agency dialogue with the wider state/citizen relationship. At present, there seems little prospect of any official encouragement of such work. It seems clear from the plans for reorganising NHS institutions set out in such documents as *A first class service* (NHS Executive, 1998) that, although a number of new initiatives related to user involvement have been taken, the underlying model of control of the health care arena is still one of hierarchy rather than network: of government rather than governance.

References

Alford, R.R. and Friedland, R. (1985) *Powers of theory: Capitalism, the state and democracy*, Cambridge: Cambridge University Press.

Audit Commission (1992) *Community care: Managing the cascade of change*, London: HMSO.

Barnes, C. and Oliver, M. (1995) 'Disability rights: rhetoric and reality in the UK', *Disability and Society*, vol 10, no 1, pp 111-16.

Barnes, M. and Prior, D. (1995) 'Spoilt for choice? How consumerism can disempower public service users', *Public Money and Management*, vol 15, no 3, pp 53-8.

Barnes, M. and Shardlow, P. (1996) 'Identity crisis? Mental health user groups and the "problem" of identity', in C. Barnes and G. Mercer (eds) *Exploring the divide: Illness and disability*, Leeds: The Disability Press.

Barnes, M. and Wistow, G. (1991) *Changing relationships in community care*, Working Paper No 3, Leeds: University of Leeds Nuffield Institute for Health.

Barnes, M. and Wistow, G. (1994) *User oriented community care: An overview of findings from an evaluation of the Birmingham Community Care Special Action Project*, Leeds: University of Leeds Nuffield Institute for Health.

Barnes, M., Harrison, S., Mort, M., Shardlow, P. and Wistow. G. (1996) *Consumerism and citizenship amongst users of health and social care services*, Project no L311253025, End of Award Report to ESRC.

Barnes, M., Harrison, S., Mort, M., Shardlow, P. and Wistow, G. (1998) 'The new management of community care: user self-organisation and co-production', in G. Stoker (ed) *The new management of local governance: Hierarchy, markets and networks*, Basingstoke: Macmillan.

Cooper, L., Coote, A., Davies, A. and Jackson, C. (1995) *Voices off: Tackling the democratic deficit in health*, London: Institute for Public Policy Research.

Coote, A. and Lenaghan, J. (1997) *Citizens' juries: Theory into practice*, London: Institute for Public Policy Research.

Dalton, R. J. and Kuechler, M. (eds) (1990) *Challenging the political order: New social and political movements in western democracies*, Cambridge: Polity Press.

Davey, B. (1994) *Empowerment through holistic development: A framework for egalitarianism in the ecological age*, Nottingham: Nottingham Advocacy Group/Ecoworks.

Davey, B. (1999) 'Solving economic, social and environmental problems together: an empowerment strategy for losers', in M. Barnes and L. Warren (eds) *Paths to empowerment,* Bristol: The Policy Press.

Department of Health (1990) *Community care in the next decade and beyond: Policy guidance*, London: HMSO.

Department of Health (1992) *Implementing care for people: Assessment*, CI(92)34, London: Department of Health.

Dowswell, T., Harrison, S., Mort, M. and Lilford, R.J. (1997) *Health panels: A survey*, Project No HSR015, End of Award Report to NHS Executive (Northern and Yorkshire), Leeds: University of Leeds Nuffield Institute for Health.

Ellis, K. (1993) *Squaring the circle. User and carer participation in needs assessment*, York: Joseph Rowntree Foundation.

Fox, C.J. and Miller. H.T. (1995) *Postmodern public administration: Towards discourse*, London: Sage.

Gell, C. (1987) 'Learning to lobby. The growth of patients' councils in Nottingham', in I. Barker and E. Peck (eds) *Power in strange places. User empowerment in mental health services*, London: Good Practices in Mental Health.

Harrison, S. (1991) 'Working the markets: purchaser/provider separation in English health care', *International Journal of Health Services*, vol 21, no 4, pp 625-36.

Harrison, S., Barnes, M. and Mort, M. (1997) 'Praise and damnation: mental health user groups and the construction of organisational legitimacy', *Public Policy and Administration*, vol 12, no 2, pp 4-16.

Heater, D. (1990) *Citizenship: The civic ideal in world history, politics and education*, London: Longman.

Hirschman, A.O. (1970) *Exit, voice and loyalty*, Cambridge MA: Harvard University Press.

Keat, R., Whiteley, N. and Abercrombie, N. (eds) (1994) *The authority of the consumer*, London: Routledge.

King's Fund (1980) *An ordinary life*, Project Paper 24, London: King's Fund.

Knox, C. and McAlister, D. (1995) 'Policy evaluation: incorporating users' views', *Public Administration*, vol 73, no 3, pp 413-16.

Lindow, V. and Morris, J. (1995) *Service user involvement. Synthesis of findings and experience in the field of community care*, York: Joseph Rowntree Foundation.

Lovenduski, J. and Randall, V. (1993) *Contemporary feminist politics*, Oxford: Oxford University Press.

Marshall, T.H. (1950) *Citizenship and social class and other essays*, Cambridge: Cambridge University Press.

Meehan, E. (1993) 'Citizenship and the European Community', *Political Quarterly*, vol 64, no 2, pp 172-86.

NHS Executive (1995) *Priorities and planning guidance for the NHS: 1996/97*, London: HMSO.

NHS Executive (1998) *A first class service: Quality in the new NHS*, London: Department of Health.

NHSME (NHS Management Executive) (1992) *Local voices. The views of local people in purchasing for health*, London: Department of Health.

Plant, R. (1992) 'Citizenship, rights and welfare', in A. Coote (ed) *The welfare of citizens*, London: Rivers Oram Press.

Pollitt, C. (1993) *Managerialism and the public services*, Oxford: Blackwell.

Prior, D., Stewart, J. and Walsh, K. (1995) *Citizenship: Rights, community and participation*, London: Pitman.

Raadschelders, J.C.N. (1995) 'Rediscovering citizenship: historical and contemporary reflections', *Public Administration*, vol 73, no 4, pp 611-25.

Ranson, S. and Stewart, J. (1994) *Management for the public domain*, Basingstoke: Macmillan.

Rhodes, R.A.W. (1997) *Understanding governance: Policy networks, governance, reflexivity and accountability*, London: Sage.

Roche, M. (1992) *Rethinking citizenship: Welfare, ideology and change in modern society*, Cambridge: Polity Press.

Secretaries of State (1989) *Caring for people: Community care in the next decade and beyond*, Cm849, London: HMSO.

Secretary of State for Health (1997) *The new NHS: Modern, dependable*, Cm3807, London: The Stationery Office.

Stewart, J. (1992) *Accountability to the public*, London: European Policy Forum.

Towell, D. (ed) (1988) *An ordinary life in practice*, London: King's Fund.

Tudor Hart, J. (1994) *Feasible socialism: The National Health Service, past, present and future*, London: Socialist Health Association.

Twine, F. (1994) *Citizenship and social rights: The interdependence of self and society*, London: Sage.

van der Male, R. (1995) 'Clientmovement in Europe: its past, present and future', *Psychiatria et Neurologia Japonica*, vol 97, no 7, pp 517-21.

Williams, P. and Schoultz, B. (1984) *We can speak for ourselves*, Bloomington: Indiana University Press.

Wistow, G. and Hardy, B. (1994) 'Community care planning', in N. Malin (ed) *Implementing community care*, Buckigham: Open University Press.

Wolfensberger, W. (1972) *The principle of normalisation in human service*, Toronto: National Institute of Mental Retardation.

Wood, B. (forthcoming) *Patient power? Patients' associations in Britain and America*, Buckingham: Open University Press.